The hands are a majestic tool! The feet are the mirror of our soul. Effectiveness of the immune system depends on the amount of electricity being magnified by the heart, and the ability of the brain to prepare orders. Naturally, the imbalances which make us unique, are because no one can truly feel the meaning behind own inner pain. We ultimately decide our own destiny. The work it takes to mold ourselves into professional athletes is so vast, that we call the few who succeed superstars. Without our own hands in the dirt, lifting up our knees to hit the turf, without our own effort to breathe, to look where we are landing and step with the toes; we are doomed and bound to sickness. The skill of manually turning bones and skins, and forcefully twisting muscles and joints, is the art of Acupressure.

Our body, mind and soul play equal parts in the search for health, but neither is attainable in their full capacity without physical health. Proper reflections of electrical signals to the body, must reroute themselves back up from the ground, in order for the heart and the brain to retain their original signature and integrity. If the mind and soul are twisted, so will be our bodies and actions, and if the body is sick, vice versa. As age catches up with our youth, the knee caps, the sacral, the stomach, the head and the spinal column twist inward; all the other joints and muscles twist left or right. All aspects of our lives slow down proportionally, as our bodies become stiff and disabled; we often don't see the marks in the state of our mental and spiritual health until it's too late. The mind has been operated by numerous surgeons, and the soul has been influenced by many churches. Only the muscles and the bones can be logically untwisted, and corrected. I believe that all thoughts and feelings must be in harmony with the body for someone to truly be healthy, and the only door that is clearly open is through physical health. I know from personal experience that our body can be re-aligned to move accordingly, as we command with our mind and soul. Acupressure is the ancient art of sports medicine which allows a complete makeover of the human body, while brushing on the mind and soul.

If judge not unless you are judging yourself is the highest teachings in spiritual terms, then knowledge with no limits would fit for intellectuality and wisdom beyond for athletes in physical health. This world of mechanical body motion that I lose myself in, is an ancient mystery school of math, astronomy, and medicine; where work was working on us, to achieve the highest possibility of our gift as human. Something unstoppable is pulling the right side to the ground, you have no choice but to bring the left down with it to accommodate, gravity is unavoidable. With our own hands, we would sculpture our bodies and those of our youth; in our minds, we intended goodness to be the law. Each joint and each muscle group must be manually unwrapped; tolerance and patience would also be accompanied by scientific notebooks. This Egyptian institution created pharaohs, and forced labor; with the intention to build kings, not slaves! Who became the masters? The wanted to teach their own perception of the truth behind the purpose of creation; these powerful thinkers decided to use partly the truth to direct a population's minds to their advantage. Acupressure disappeared as a whole and became religion. The hands, the thoughts and the feet became lost in the world of economics. Health has become a second priority to utilization and profit. God cannot be one person! Intellectuality cannot be the highest strength of mankind.

I was always the odd ball who did not want my close friends to know that I wear glasses and loved biology. Hardly interested in school, but basketball and girls kept I motivated. What I really wanted, I did not know what it was; how can I find the place to look? I will recognize a humble person when I meet one; in my heart I can feel it. I have chosen myself to conceive the Holy Spirit; I am not looking for approval? I knew the teachings of man have grown in the opposite side of goodness, with education that's lethal. I must learn from the mistakes and breakthroughs of all others whom have trod this land in the name of righteousness, to enrich myself with their wisdom and knowledge. Why is man such an animal? Why am I not so vain? Whatever happened to our mind, body and soul; I will try to fix it!

The head is a simultaneous 12 way calculate, solve, transmit, receive, nuclear reactor. When the feet are hitting the ground properly; they are 12 signals that enter the body at -10+2. The +2 are harvested by the fingers are always presents, but the -10 can only manifest if the feet are grounded. If the head is a 1=12, equal to the opposite of the feet at -10, than the thorax cannot be a 12 in relation to the cervical spine at 7, the thorax may be a 6 when there is circular movement between R7-8. With the lumbar at 5, and the sacral/coccyx at -5+4.The thorax has breaks between T3-4 and

T7-8 to make it a 3, 4, 5 segment. The way the legs coil around R12-11, to the other side of R8-7, the spinal column cannot be twisted in just one direction. In fact the Coccyx and C7 would turn to the opposite with at least one vertebra in the thorax would be leaning left. Dexter Scoliosis has been teaching me the reasons why the body gets old and sick and disable. Too much pain, a child must be guided; it is my duty to teach the youth how to stay fit!

My own head has been pounding from multiple concussions. My shoulders had my neck by the throat and the scapula was playing poppet pull on my thorax and on my sternum. I could see a bulge on my left rib cage, stopping circular movement at R8, 9, 10. I could not bend too far on the right side of my stomach; it felt as if there was a hole on the middle quadrant. All my weight rested on the left Iliac; I knew it was where the right leg rotation was stocked. My left knee had a contusion; my right knee cap was playing drums with the meniscus, my left heel was having competition with my right big toe; every part of my body were taking their turns at paining, and teaching me their proper positioning. I am so lucky, I've been gifted with the ability to feel the muscles, and know which way to push or pull them back into their original location. I had the perfect body to learn every inch of the human body; as mine was completely damaged.

This is my journey on a road that has become a myth, when Earth was healthy, and there was an obligatory medical school, to teach all human how to heal themselves. I bet, all information that once existed has been duplicated in our genes, and areas of interest have a memory bank in our subconscious. I will use stories, essays, poems and songs to take you with me on a trip towards health. I write in mainly English, but overall I will communicate with you in four languages. I will sincerely try to enlighten you with my knowledge of the human body. Our minds and souls are unique, so pardon my self-expression, if and when I hit you with a twist.

A strange feeling that is, when sugar enters in a cavity; it aches in a way that says quickly, Tylenol3. That's just a small aspect of the constant turbulence and chaos happening inside our bodies, but yet those chemical reactions are our life form force and energy. What a painful way to describe our existence; the only solution is accept this truth, God is a mad scientist! Is it really understandable, why mankind is so crazy; yet we are God's most unique, perfect creation! This guy needs to stay out of the lab, seriously! Our body works with acute electrical pulses and crossed weight pressure, on nervous muscular contractions.

Sometimes I feel that my left side is responsible for my physical impairment, but no, I think it's my right side causing all the problems the next day. I love this side of me that is innovative and a champion athlete. Damn, is that also me, as I looked in the mirror across my head? The same stories in the news are reenacting in my mind; here is the bigger problem, underneath my own scalp. The two sides must work together, I must control right and wrong, good and bad; that's how the body works the best. The reaction of stomach acids and oxygen on the food gives us energy in blood. The friction of our muscles around the ribs and the nerves gives electricity to our brain through our heart. C7 process it all. All these parts together, make us function like such wonderful beings some days, and as not so adorable children others.

Understanding the nature of God may not always be believable! A dog showed me how to sweep my feet and roll. A cat taught me how to lift my left leg and jump. A baby boy showed me how to sit down; my step daughter taught me how to stretch my hips. My son showed me how to stretch my back; my daughter taught me how to stretch my chest. I had told God that if he wanted to teach me, he's going to have to do it himself; so he gave me a beautiful daughter. Dear God, I have never loved this way before. I have never been so protective of anyone like I body guard my princess Melanie! She has taught me to cool down my voice, to ignore, to move on, and to keep on! She forgets so quickly, she has helped me to see that this world is always on the news with another headline to keep us confused, and not to let it affect me too much in my moods. Do girls learn how to spend people's money in the tummy? That's $700.00 she just made me spend in 55 minutes, at 10 years old! We're not going back to the mall anytime soon. I have also learned that God has been preparing me to heal Earth all along, as something inside of me has been teaching me how to heal myself, so I can one day help others. Until I have given it my best shot, than I don't believe anything is impossible. Dexter Scoliosis is simply my university; it isn't an incurable disease alike in the diagnosis given to me by modern medicine

. When walking or running, the steps start on the toes, use both hands equally. Walk and run alike going up and downstairs, or like jumping rope, in a straight line, while counting 1, 2, 3; to switch sides, and breathe every other 3. An angel's steps start with the left foot. This hypothesis which changes our present way of walking around the world is the key towards a healthy body. Walking the wrong way, starting our steps on the heels as we do today, is the beginning cause of all chronic diseases known to our civilized society, and the sole destroyer of our immune system. I am challenging Harvard University, and all others in the circle of high class influential medical studies. We need to bring this subject to Capitol Hill! First and foremost, I need to heal myself! My belief is only an illusion if I only know the theory on paper, and unable to untwist the Thorax; I would only be a modern day doctor.

It's so clear to me that the body should land on the toes, like when going down the stairs. Why can't others see that, the way they walk has everything to do with their state of health? Guess I've got to show them. Look at me now! Do you love me? I can dance! I've been working on myself for so long! I feel as if I am getting so strong! I've got to get there! No excuses! I am going to Zion! Have you ever felt so good, so high, that you could sing with bobby in the clouds, touching the sky over the falling rain; I mean jump over the hurdles of life? I can see the light, underneath the rocks in the tunnel! I'm almost there! Where am I? This is so dark! Creator, are you there? You know these people don't believe me right! They're laughing at me saying, he's walking like a girl! Boy! This side is closed! How did you get in here? You were not supposed to come through the light! God! Somebody came in here through the back! Malice, where is Mother Earth? Ginette! Somebody's looking for you! Hey son! Hurry child go! Father is coming! When walking or running, the steps start with the toes! Are you serious, is that it? An angel's step starts with the left foot! Okay! Fly like a dragon, fly! Fast! Say, father I'm a sinner, when you see him! I'm a singer! No, say Jah I have sinned! They say I have sung in the English grammar madre! Hello queen! Jehovah! Hi! Stop! Hey you! Help! Help! Array! Father, I'm a sinner, I sing, I sung, I have sinned, why have you forsaken me? Sorry, forgive me, I love you. I'm only human, thought you'd left me. This hurts! Dude, you're calling people crazy, and you're the God who created them; while you' re letting them stick people with needles and nails crucified them on a cross, shooting them with electrical current and bullets, to watch them die! You are insane! Aren't you the judge? Who the xxxx you're talking to kid? I was wondering if my visions were just an illusion, whether my belief in you is just another delusion, God. O, we got ourselves a smarty pants hey, how about you go back to Earth the same way you got here, and go learn how to speak politely! I don't know how I got here! Excuse me sir, I can't fly, I can't fly, I can't fly! Is it just my arrogance stating that I would heal myself from this pain lingering inside of me in my body, head and soul, with your help? The same pain that has tormented every living being on this planet! Is that how it can be beaten? Yes! Are you sure 100% yes? When walking or running, the steps start with the toes! Yes! It sounds too simple. Use both sides equally! They are other parts involved like always, when you read the fine prints.

It took me a century it seems to even feel how the spring pump actually operates, when you walk the right way; and how walking the wrong way could truly mess up, everything up stream. Prior to that day, when the left heel started hurting, before the left ankle got loose, and the hips re-balanced to a workable angle; my body was so broken up that even I had doubt in myself. Why can't people see that this is it? In my head, during the 17 years that I remained silent to study the human body, I intended to re-educate the world as soon as my health reflected greatness against the shiniest stars. Yeah! My left ankle is loosening up for real. I could feel the spring motion of the amazing foot. I've finally been able to lift the right knee; than the hip ball rolled up, giving way for me to move the pelvic girdle. After the gluteus Maximus was partially re-aligned and the sacral was receiving stronger signals from the hip, my brain has been able to re-calculate and fix everything in its route; even my vision stopped being blurry, my headaches and muscle pain are also retreating slowly. This pain feels so good, as my spine started to spin freer; I became surer of my hypothesis which God had given to me as a present for my insolence. They told me, when walking or running, the steps start on the toes and to use both hands equally.

I've been able to push up and to the left on the lumbar L5 to T1 in the thorax, and continue up from C7 to C1, to where the carotid meets with the occipital bone. That tilt of the upper spinal column which appears to be to the left in the thorax is the common maladies found in older folks as the body age; it is caused by a pull at T8, from the left shoulder, due to misused. Although this last deformation looks to be on to the left for people who are right handed; the spinal column is actually twisted to the right. The hips must be balanced before attempting to untwist the thorax. Although I knew what to do, and how to do it; not being able to reach my own back with both hands, to apply enough pressure, put another tweak in my journey. But with work and perseverance, day by day, my health is getting better and better. I had to write and inform the world of a new day that has begun. To achieve health one must walk and run, starting the steps on the toes.

I’ve taken that turn so many times. Is this confusion hills already? It seems as if every time I get close to completion level, something drags me down. What is it that is really stopping me? That same ankle again, or is it the shoulder this time? I was just so happy and confident a minute ago, why am I feeling so blue all of a sudden? Is it the physical pain, or the mental strain?

My back started hurting badly after my girl left me. Maybe, oh! Baby, don’t say that! I need you! I do have faith, I can please you! All night long, until the break of dawn! Is that your Louis Vuitton purse? I got enough to quench your thirst! Thank you so much for the quick rent comes first! It’s been 3 months; I haven’t seen a night nurse! Do I believe in God? Yes I do, but this is not a good time right now, can I get back to you St Pierre, whoever you are talking to me in my head all the time. Let me tell you the truth, I’ve already paid her; do you understand English! Who is God? I am, right now according to her! You are too, you could be, and we are! Wait, I don’t think we have the same definition of God! Small detail, you need to see that guy up front at the gulches, to pay like everybody else in this dungeon. Alright now, someone saying that they have good intentions, that they strive to do it godly, does not grant them crucifixion! You've ask me a question, so I've answered. I've got to go! Mr. Christ! So, you are the creator? No, I did not create heaven and Earth. I did not create mankind! She just sparked the joint I rolled up; can we do a thirty minute break without prayer? I've heard stories from the Bible about a guy named Jesus! What you criminals did to that man was wrong; you did not even give him a chance to explain. Can you put the busy sign on the door this time Simon? St. Joseph, can you hear me now? Good for you, you've got universal coverage! Ok, no one is home right now. Is there an angel talking? Nanananananana! I've suffered enough pain already. I'm not trying to die and get up to prove that I am God. That is not a test anyone can pass. God is in our actions as we are alive! God is all creation! Resurrection to me is reviving this dead body that you're walking with. Reincarnation is a long turn around the Galaxy! I'm okay with hell right now. I got a little bit of money to pay taxes to Caesar! No, I don't want to go to heaven. Not the place you're calling Wet Sand! I almost got stocked there, I don't wanna pray all day. I just got a new girlfriend waiting for me inside; Babylon is being good to me right now! Do you like me at all; would you please come back later?

I must go back to feeling invincible like when I was 14. After I had made a wish to become a priest at the age of 7; a dark cloud had started to follow me, digging pot holes on my road. It all turned dark one day. I was born perfect; it's only the teachings of this world that has rotten my thoughts. Alike every other child born on this Earth, we all pay the price for bad parenting. Blame it on somebody else isn't that human nature?

The laws of nature, as we know it, say that death is the wages of sin! What is a sin? A sin is anything you do to destroy the body, mind or soul. Is having sex a sin? Did Eve bite the apple? Did Adam hit brown sugar? Wrong spot! Don't stop! Oh, you like that! They call that rug burns from the doggy style! I don't think God is going to be too happy with us picking apples today. Eve, its broad day light! Come on Adam we'll just tell him it was for pro-creation studies. We both agreed, well, did you enjoy it? Physical interaction is a needed part of life, as long as there's acceptance. So no I don't think sexing too much would make God close the door on us and make our lives a living hell.

What about not going to school, being illiterate, is that a sin? HSD, GED, BAC, MD, PHD, that's too many acronyms. Do you mean if someone is non-conformant to the standards of this society, is that a sin? No, if you are a pirate of the Caribbean, your chansonette in the passing zone is F…. Caesar…K...Caesar…R…Caesar, all these dots are bad words against obedience. You don't need to know how to read or write to be smart, you do need to know how to count your money though, and then you're good to go. Alain, stop it! No sir! The intellectual portion of the brain must be developed also to fully appreciate life. Pirates do need to tell which direction is home without hitting a rock island. However, ABC's and 123's are not logically the first things we should teach children to focus on. Their physical health and morals should cover all the younger years until they can remember instructions on the right way to walk, and maintain descent habits and postures at the dinner table.

We are all unique, even if the majority thinks a certain way; they are always exceptions to any rule. So what is an example of a sin, what is the original sin? The silent assassin is the heels! Walking on the heels destroys the body so bad; that the brain thinks it is okay to bomb people, in the name of a holy war, and claim to have love in the heart, that is in God we trust that the embargo will crush them all! I believe that walking on the heels is the original sin, because all kids start their steps on the toes to stand the first time; before the age of 3, they all will start to walk on their heels. They are some exceptions of kids who keep on walking on their toes from birth; that is also an abnormality which is diagnosed as having some type of mental disability, which I think is physically triggered. It is bad for the heels to be stock up or down. The heels must be able to move up and down for the transfer of energy to happen fully between the symphysis pubis, the Xiphoid and the sacrum.

So here we are mixing God with medicine. They say that he was a scientist and a healer! Yo! Homeboy, I need some help here! Alike any other person in extreme pain, I was asking God, "Why do I cry these tears from my eyes, why must I carry this heavy, heavy load?" (Tosh), cursing at God for allowing man to hurt my body so badly. Thanking him at the same time for choosing me, to show the greatness of his majesty. I would not have figured out how to fix most parts of my body, without the other side being broken, dislocated or jammed.

Evil thoughts were not going to sit there and just let goodness easily take over its righteous place in my mind, body or soul. Of course the devils had instructions to all legions, stop anyone from passing through its gates heading towards good living land! I knew that there was no way all doors could be closed. Just like a bad thief always leaves a trace, there has got to be a flaw. I'm writing because I want to help humanity feel better. Now all over is sickness and war. Why is it that every time I felt the breeze, a storm came to crash the party. I knew that there's always a leap hole in any coups d'état. If Satan could trick God, he could also get tricked! What did he do, how did he do it? Did he make people believe some things were good, when they were actually bad? What were the different items involved? I will find them! I just need to ask enough questions. I've got to free their minds from bondage, so they can think to at least analyze before finalizing. I know one way that isn't right at all, and that is dying. People think they're going to find heaven after that! Can I keep his watch? Dying is no good man! I've never seen any dead man talk and tell anyone that they're enjoying themselves out there! We can put an X on that route! I need to look for the keys to life now, while alive.

My best friend broke my right ankle in a friendly soccer game. That big toe was already jammed. I twisted my spine in a friendly basketball game while in the U.S Navy. I dislocated my right hip playing friendly soccer, in front of the naval base in San Diego. A Tonton Macoute hit me with an oozy and broke one of my ribs. Somebody shot me in the stomach and the leg, I still don't know who, when and where it happened; I just see the bullet marks. I broke one more rib in a friendly boxing sparing match. I dislocated my right shoulder and jammed my left knee when I fell from a bike. I overextended my right knee and jammed my neck during a car accident. I got a head concussion from stupidly playing friendly tackle football with no pads. I'm forgetting a machete hit on the left tibia, and so many other sports and fighting injuries, too many to mention all of them. What friends are for? A part of my life felt like I had tweaked my finger on the spindle of a spinning wheel; as if I was cursed at birth by a malfeasant. Magically, all that had happened to me were battling my birth defect which had deformed my spine.

Nothing, no one will stop me from making it to the NBA. I must show these fools what I'm made of. I am the baldest natty dread! Don't you know that I got a playboy bunny on my right arm, made on sunset strip in Hollywood, at the joint close to the house of blues? I used to date a bunny back in my A days you know! Shoot, I'm not done! My body would not let me stay on my high horse for long. My spine was slowly degrading along with every other part of me. There has got to be a potion, a remedy, magic, a gene to help me reconnect the spinal column.

Is it okay if I smoke some marijuana God? Yupp, it makes me feel good! I'm feeling Iry, even with the pain Jah! I could feel that the hypothesis was working in my body, when walking or running the steps start on the toes; but I could also feel that it was going to be a long way from home. Marijuana and God, are we talking about Mr. Marley or King Solomon here. You know they found an ounce of good weed in his tomb. This is some high grade buds, ooh oui, these white boys got that indo down to the science; I'm loving it! Humboldt County! THC has the same structure as chemicals naturally secreted by the brain. The creative and meditative attributes of cannabis are its most known usage; I'm also trying to introduce its muscle relaxing, and bone regenerating capabilities. I know that God help those who help themselves. I don't think it would be possible to pull on my spinal vertebras, or on my skull tissue without some anesthetic help. Thank you God for the Cali for Nia, (weed for a purpose). That's right, I don't know how we let Washington and Colorado legalize marijuana before us; that's a lot of business we're losing, stop fronting. Let's get on the ball California, and legalize the weed. Jamaica and Puerto Rico are now legal too! Most people who are against marijuana are alcoholics, tobacco smokers, pill takers, ignorant posers, sexual and religious addicts, I got more, but wait. I have ordered the first commandment, when walking or running, the steps start with the toes; here's the second, thou shall put marijuana in your diet. Is this a comedy? Who's writing this, Eddie? No! I hope you like bad jokes. I am telling you to pack the chalice, light it and burn it up, pass it around this way please. We all have an opinion. Everything I say is for you to analyze, not to take for granted or final truth!

All laws have exceptions. Even with thy shall not kill; if you walk in my house unwelcomed and I think you're there to hurt me or my family; may the lord bless you for the exceptional reception I will give to you. Why be so harsh on immigrants, and call yourself American? Don't you know the history of our rebellion that made us an empire state? Why are you so mad? A thief stealing from thieves isn't that what it boils down to. I'm not talking about you cousin, you need to put that down! If you're here to steal my stuff that I worked hard for; Moses, zap, come get this guy! I do keep a baseball bat, as one of the jewels in my culture. As is with all rules in nature, there's always a better or worst way to turn it and twist it to our advantage. Why would the status quo which is killing the mass slowly, but making great profit with medication sales, be a subject of change for politicians? They, who have financial implication in the health care system, are the main reason for malpractice in medicine.

They are always trials, errors and lessons learnt from mistakes. Could walking on the heels be a big mistake of our ignorance? Are we being kept from information that could help us heal ourselves? Were we force do as told? Is it too late to prepare for better trading laws? Are the majority of rulers doing it for wrong? Check a mango for worms before you eat it! Because insulin can help stabilize diabetes, it doesn't mean a child needs to get it. I do believe that there is a higher power guiding and leading us to sickness and death, and it's called government. This world which had also once made a believer out of me, that the grave in the cemetery was my only opportunity.

Come into the light with me and seek health as the precious stone. We can design our own destiny if we are healthy! I cannot let the children go through such pain. As bad as I felt my spine and head were before my spring pumps became operative; I know that I've been mystically kept alive, I am blessed. If only you knew how sick your body was, you would give thanks and praises 3 times a day like a Muslim, just to stretch or to say thanks to Allah. Did I get it right? Is it Jehovah witnesses? No, they're the ones who knock on the door during football Sunday. God is not welcome right now man, we're going all out; we got Gogo girls, beers, weed, alcohol and spicy barbecued ribs and chicken. Is that girl with you; does she go to your church? Come in, come in! Okay, I'll go play with you, I mean pray. Do Rastas pray? Oh yeah, that's my kind of religion; I want to be there when the smoking. No matter if you are Caucasian, African, Latin or Asian; all kids should eat in a home with education, sing songs of happiness, and grow into great human beings. By teaching our kids to walk, starting their steps with their toes, we will guarantee for them a healthy future.

The foot is a spring pump that works when our body weight lands on the toes. The foot is also an electrical ground. The heels do touch the ground in the middle of the rotation, except when sprinting. This amazing aspect of the foot that I found, after years of pounding on my toes; I believe is the single most important preventive medicine discovery of modern day. If the foot, which is our foundation, has faulty lines, there is no chance to build a strong body on such stones. The immune system which works directly with the condition of our electrical system is weakened tremendously from walking on the heels. A shed can be wiped away by a thunderstorm, not a fortress. They are so many lives being lost due to our selfishness, cruelty and ignorance. While walking with the heels first, like we are accustoming to, even the pictures in the biology book that we use to teach our children are deformed. All the examples we have today are all of people who walked on their heels. Without this ability of the heel to separate smoothly from the ankle and move up and down, left and right; every joint in the body will have a problem.

After the feet are stretched, the hips can be rebalanced manually by pulling on the pelvic girdle and the Iliac. The hip balls can also be manually taught to roll. The knees don't get to work properly until the feet and the hips are set. The big toes are largely responsible for the state of knees. The ankles control the ability of R8 to slide under R7. The fingers have great effects on elbows and the cervical spine. The wrists control the ability of R3 to move off the sternum. The weak side must be retrained and fine-tuned alike the writing hand. There is one line from R1, to the scapula, to R8 that remains connected to the spinal column, pulling on muscles of the neck and thorax; as long as there is an imbalance. Up front on that same left arms, muscles of shoulder also attach themselves to R1 and the chess cage; pulling on ribs casing the heart. There are so many problems that are caused by walking the wrong way and not using both hands.

This is a thesis and a challenge to all medical authorities, doctors of the world, trainers, coaches, etc. Stop lying to the people, stop practicing surgery on them, stop prescribing them pills, you cannot heal them. I am calling you out. I wish to discuss debate, demonstrate and compete against the status quo, which encourages people to continue walking with their heels hitting the ground first. I wish to erase the hypocrisy within the medical society, and re-polish what's left with my hypothesis which states: when walking or running, the steps start with the toes, use both sides equally. "Emancipate yourselves from mental slavery, none but our self can free our own mind." (Marley)

There is no health without running. All muscular and joint pain is due to the irregular rotation of the body from waking the wrong way. Most chronic diseases, like hypertension, cancer, scoliosis, etc., also take roots from the lack of perfusion created by deformations from walking the wrong way. The movement always starts with the ring toe (it works together as one with the small toe, to the heels, and rolling off the big toe. The other two toes feel as middle men and work equally with the proximate toe. While sprinting, the steps may start straight on the big toe to push and glide.

The magic spirit did not arrive for me until the 5th day of Christmas, when everything moved like a left hander. The right toe, left knee, right hip, left shoulder, right ear, than the joint at T12, T8 and L5 realigned partially. My left ankle had started to spring a few of months earlier, and I had pulled on the pelvic girdle and the Iliac to partly rebalance my hips. Than I thought I was ready to raw for 12 rounds of boxing like a lion, full court one on one anyone basketball, football, futbol, hockey, one hundred meter dash. Not yet, said the headaches. Don't you know there are bills to pay and baby mamas in the script?

Am I going to be the first to regain elasticity? I will work until my last breath, if it is to keep my dignity. It took me years to over shadow my own doubts; so naturally I looked at the saying, that it is impossible to change City Hall, as dreadful not unmanageable. How hard could it be to reach Washington? I need the President and Congress to help me institutionalized this new way worldwide. When walking or running, the steps start with the toes.

In 2001, my spinal injury was diagnosed as being incurable. I'm the kind of kid who still believes in Santa Claus. Hey King, where is Chrystal's globe? Can I take a look? I can't see anything. O well, I'm proceeding blindly, like a train going down hills with no breaks, with my attempt to talk to you and tell you again and again; when walking or running, the steps start with the toes. Even though I know I might hit another cold wall, I hope there's another escape route to reach you. I must try to convince you with this vision I have of being the chosen one to make the future on Earth a pleasant stay. By fixing our body, our mind and soul will be able to function properly; we would be able to stop all the wars, and apply true diplomacy.

Are we living in a democratic society? Is the meaning of democracy the cut version of theocracy, sizzled to accommodate the rich in power? Are there any good governments? Did I answer your question? We would be more thoughtful of our neighbors and their needs if we were healthy. There would be no children hungry if we were a super power. They are 675 million hungry people every day. Yes we can make a difference in the world. We all must take the lead for the protection of Justice and fairness. Who am I kidding? Each one of us must show the world that we are the glue that brings all creation together somehow, in the name of goodness! So,what do you want to do today Dick? I do want some of that oil money from Haiti G. What are you talking about; I thought they only had gold? Let's take over the world B! I was whispering OB! The walls can hear us in here Chelle! All sails up, full speed ahead, sonar, radar, radio, navigation, torpedo room, launch! Hit, we got them, they signed the license, the gold rush is on, hurry, hurry, it's on! As poor as these people are already; stealing from them is not just a crime, it is inhumane. You are pitiful thieves.

Being poor and unlucky is a way of conceiving a rich life as being materially stable and married. Poorly educated however, is a guaranteed failure, that's being poor! Modern medicine teaches us that the spinal column makes a wall with the Iliac. The sacral is supposed to move slightly inversely, with the movements of the spinal column; it is not supposed to be a big block with the hips. They are fused to the sacral only because the balls can't roll when the ankles are locked, to allow the hips to complete the rotation and move freely to remain aligned with the spinal column. When walking with the heels first as the status quo teaches; it is impossible for the ankles to disconnect properly from the foot like when jumping up, or landing from a dunk. If the symphysis pubis is affected by the imbalance, the pelvic girdle would be too. A group of muscles harden to limit any circular or up and down movement that may cause nerves from the sacral to touch the hip wall. Any small miss alignment between the symphysis pubis and the sacrum would cause energy transfer to slowly diminish its possible output. It is impossible to align the spine without the sacral being spaced symmetrically inside the hips. After the feet are loose, the pelvic girdle must be manually pulled back across the right line by forcefully pulling on the Gluteus Maximus. These same aspects between the Sacral and the hips are duplicated between the Xiphoid and R8, 9, 10; the only difference is that the muscles of the stomach don't get hard, they widen.

The body is made of 4 strange circles rotating around a bending, conductive electrical rod, and sitting on a mechanical spring! The legs and the arms connect between R8, R7. A cross pattern permits the left leg to work with the right shoulder ant the left brain; on top of the right leg which is attached to the heart and the creative side of our brain. Once the sacral is exactly in the middle of the hips, and the pumps in the feet are helping with pumping blood back up; you could be as light as Sugar Ray and as heavy as metal, because there will be amplification within the spinal cord.

The misused of one side is a major player in our sick living and causes further complications in energy transfer to the sternum and spinal column, added to walking the wrong way. For people who write with their right hand and leave their left hand unused; the lack of fine tuning of the weak side causes muscles belonging to that shoulder to stiffen and limit motion of the thorax, the cervical spine and sternum. This protective ability of the skin and muscles to become hard between joints and limit movement can be reversed by manually re-separating the muscle groups affected, after the obstructions give way.

The barriers that took me faraway west, were the edgy road with a chance to grow into myself, and develop the vision I've had of a place they called Earth the paradise, not just Jamaica! I had been searching for love. The kind of caring that is able to provide bread and butter for his soldiers, perfume and spice for his queens. I want to show you how much I love you by putting myself on the spot of a new research, to prove that when walking or running the steps start with the toes, and to use both sides equally.

Loving God, I've learnt that it takes patience, forgiveness and tolerance to love. Isn't that a B; they're calling each other, sending gifts and going to mass; and I'm right here. Guess they don't see me that way. Am I not a special creation of God? I am part of he and he is me! I had been a bad boy for too long, none of my high school friends and family would believe that I went godly. They must not know how having a beautiful daughter can change a vagabond into a father, preacher.

It was the winter of 98, in Boston Massachusetts, over my auntie's house, in the addict where I used to dose. Maybe it was the Ste. Ides, or maybe it was smoke from the El Producto filled up with Hay. I had a dream. In it, I went to see God, and because of my arrogance, he sent me back to Earth, stating that

Satan can go ahead and keep me in hell, that I was too dangerous to enter heaven. My mother did not agree, she laughed, but my father knew what he was doing. God always have a plan, even when everything is obscure in our sight. I intended to be God's soldier, and wanted to battle the wicked at his home. This is not a war of machines at all; this is happening inside of me. Inside of you is the biggest struggle between good and evil. No one has yet broken the gates of death. Old age and sickness has had its way and made fools out of intellectuals, scientists and believers. So why should we stop this fast speed train, knowing it's on a disparaging path, and get back on our choo-choo train?

I've been at almost untwisted the spinal column, which was stamped as incurable, for the past 20 years. Nobody should have to go through so much pain. This is why I'm trying to make this hypothesis public so we may be able to prevent a painful life for our kids. I wish to physically and scientifically prove to you that the way I have discovered is the missing piece in our health puzzle. When walking or running, the steps start with the toes, use both sides equally. This is the answer to all our health questions, and it will also erase unnecessary spending on things that can be fixed with proper education.

It came to me, to try and figure out why do people commonly walk with their heels first. In the beginning stages of life, the amplification of signals is done with toes and fingers tweaks to activate the hip function and shoulder reaction. When the atmosphere changes and the ground is ground, the feet can no longer use the signature 3 coming from the mother's womb; they must feel the weight of the body on the natural ground to activate the hips. Children start to roll and crawl. They hold on to something and stand. They start to walk! They don't know why some of it hurt. They will do the most comfortable thing to survive now. They soon start to walk on their heels. Most of us try to take the easiest routes. Unless children are reminded to land accurately; they will all continue to walk on the heels towards ill health.

Instead of spending all that money on health care bills, drug abuse and rehabilitation centers; maybe we could put some in on education money. Having knowledge of electrical plants and mechanical structures is extremely helpful to understand why the heels is not the extremity of the line (the leg), in order to be a true ground; neither does the heels have the shape of a landing gear. Teaching children how to walk should be a course from K-1 to college graduate. The motion happens fast when walking the right way, with the toes first, it goes from the small/ring toe, to the heels, to the big toe. A young child can easily be fooled into thinking that the landing starts there at heel. When we look at how I do the Duncan you face, you can clearly see that the landing on the feet is with the toes first, before the do not guard me solo sweat on your forehead.

The feet control the positioning of the hips and decides 3/3 full mobility of the spinal column from the coccyx to T1. The hands control cervical spine, the upper thorax, the elbows, shoulders, clavicle and sternum.

The placement of the clavicles decides 2/3 of the spinal column's mobility from T1 to the coccyx.

The head decides 1/3 movement of cervical spine from C1 to C7, but is always added up to at least one provider of return signals. The head is the ultimate controller of the cervical spine.

The clavicles are the primary provider and can support the demands of the head to less than half its capacity.

The hips as the secondary provider must have amplification vibration coming from the feet in order to transfer to the sacral and be accepted by the brain.

Only the feet provide an electro-post strong enough to excite the spinal column fully. Every human walking on their heels are using less than 1/3 of the brain's full capacity, because their hip rotation does not start at the toes, added to the under usage of the weak side. I can remember some statistics neighboring the bottom edge of these numbers. The amount of circular motion related to the spinal column is equivalent to our state of health and electrical production. Let's use our brain. Let us teach the youth how to walk. When walking or running, the steps start with the toes.

Every single thing wrong with the human body can be associated with a bump on the head. Reflection of bodily sickness can also be found at the feet and the hands, depending on what organ being affected. Because the sternum, the spinal column and the head cannot be perfectly positioned without the feet being properly planted and the hips balanced; and because nothing works properly without the heels being able to spring up and down; I think the key to physical health is mostly at the bending of the toes. Once you understand how the body works, you too will be amazed of all its different parts. How the foot lands on the ground and the mechanism of the heel, remains as the most important foundation of a healthy body in my mind.

When I decided to carry my burden and accept my path, it was clear to me that God had plans for me, other than my wishes to be a Playboy. The pain that was in me would not let me rest, I was 28, and what do you mean incurable, Mr. Doctor? What about my ding-illing that is no longer working right and shrinking? That's not wow at all man, come on! I have many females to attend to and a reputation to maintain, this can't be! As we all find God when things go south, I too became very religiously worried. My spine was hurting nonstop, causing me pain and discomfort; but the part that got me to concentrate on regaining my health is still that thing I noticed. Jesus Christ, O Lord my savior, this is for real, I got a ruler, she remember how it used to be, my penis was getting smaller, and so was my time of explosion. Oh no, we can't have that clip in the movie, cut, that's not happening. I love God, yes I do, and his ladies too. Johnny, Johnny, wake up, up! Look at her Johnny! No don't go, No! God! What are you doing to me? Hope you understand my motivation players. She did not call me minute man, did she? No, she didn't! OMG, yes she did! My name is not Lil mini! You Venice peachy! After you've hurt my feelings, hope you're not going to ask me to borrow money for groceries anytime soon. Well, gross this! You're not funny at all saying tuth like that in public about me. I thought it was promised no talking about M or P. I better stop paying for those short sleeve T-shirts, and hide my bunny rabbit. I don't want to have to dis-satisfy anyone, anymore. I don't want to be in the hall of fame yet! No, softy is not a cool name. You got any blue pills? Those are the good ones dog, how much? Hurry up cops is coming! Don't be so paranoid! You got it bad! Man OOC since 006, caboose loose head down, finish, Don-ish, out of commission, do you understand, I need this! I shifted my energy into celibacy, parenthood and priesthood; with many prayers to Ste. Marie wishing for that thing to start working well again, please, Johnny, I'm not having much fun without you. Since you've been R.I.P, I've been lonely.

Maybe these women have a magnet, they can feel my connection is bombed and I don't many zeroes in my bank accounts. I do miss having the self-confidence to go to the club tonight with hotel keys, weed and alcohol, knowing that I'm going to score; taxi! Jimmy fits Johnny! Ooh yeah! We na go get her bumped up tonight, no. but we might rock it to the left all night long! Say words to put as lyrics in a dirty song! Well, until somebody passes out that is, we're skanking until we blow a fuse. Spark it again with the touch of love! Hold on, z-cap vroom! Plug it, shift gears, take a hit of the ease, and breathe in deep. Cough! Round two, here we go again! Come here! Change it! Yeah! Jimmy fits Johnny! Ooh yeah! Put a dry one on, than share two shots of Bacardi! We've got a recipe. We a go hit it to the right now. Looking for tight corners! What have we discovered? Second time around! This is the best hips winding round, for a brand new bang renewal. So don't be afraid to lift it up, measure it, and wait! Hit the pubis hard, like you trying to break something, than take it slow. Caress it some more, O! Don't hit the sacral! She might pack up her clothes and go! If no, than get off that channel, keep on hitting poom poom garcon. Is it on the video? Twin sister show! Off we go! Take a left on Rodeo, up the bridge to Venice beach to hustle! Going fast! Going fast! New DVDs, five dollars each, just made, five minutes ago! My brother is one of the actors, so keep it on the down low! Hopefully God and the Police are busy doing other things tonight! I also have watches, rings, ropes, incense, magazines and body oils, and if I don't have what you want on me: I can always call it in for you homie! Special delivery! Okay I'll take one of those, for support and motivation, and one of these for expression of our love, we're going to ignite fireworks. The American way!

Not appreciating the woman is a mental deprivation, a sickness! Some of these xxxxxx are crazy! What are you doing with your life if you do not love a woman? I thought I could focus on my business and my children a bit more. To explore and adore the woman on Earth is like loving the creator, who made her so beautiful. I don't have money or power; she doesn't even see me. You don't have game, I know the issue, don't be mad at me. O, I don't see you with Charlie's angels either. I thought the world was mine, and I was trying to plant my seeds everywhere the land hits the coastal. Blind, I couldn't see that the love I needed would partly be found in the kind that is associated with lust, bodily tosses and entertaining poses. I did not know than, that the sexual movements were a healthy chore. This is work! Could I get overtime? I said work is work! I will review my notes! Right now, work that back for me big momma. Tonight we're doing pelvic work out sugar, would you be my oat!

In 1998 while running on Hyde Park Avenue in December, I should have worn ice skates; because in Boston at that time of the year the sidewalks are all frozen. To stay balanced, I decided to slide like in a moon walk mode. I noticed that I was running and having fun, while watching people struggle to walk across the street to the bus stop. That same day when I got back home, I started to analyze everything that we do and realize that most athletic things we do are with the toes first: going down the stairs, jumping rope, sprinting the 100 meter dash etc. Also I noticed that all kids crawl than stand with their toes first. When I was riding the skateboard, the pain on my right hip was gone. I concluded in my head, that I needed to bring the left side down and the right side up. I wasn't sure at all that this new thing I was trying would be the beginning of my backyard medical studies.

Even though in my dream I had seen it all in the presence of God's orchestra, when Jah told me" where there's a will there's a way (Marley); my nightmares were endless and my hopes un-manifested. I had faith in heart, but the pain in my head and body made the road unbearable. To focus on the task at hand, my health, I must get rid of all these mental and emotional blockages. I'm really trying to write a theory from my hypothesis which states, when walking or running, the steps start with the toes, and so many clouds are obstructing the way. So we are clear on the picture that I'm trying to paint, and the meaning of the diagrams I'm trying to draw with words here. Don't be distracted by leafs and flowers I put around this tree to embellish this book, all parts of the process to gain health are important. I do want you to laugh and be in a pleasant mood as you read, yes; I do want you to also analyze scientifically and examine each syllable, as these words are an attempt at replacing the status quo worldwide.

I am bold, am I not? It could take both of these wanna be athletes to guard me on a football field, and I could still score a goal screaming, you need to double team me every time coach, no triple team, forget it; I want all eyes on me, do you get it. You can't keep up with me solo, pound for pound, I got you Jacked up, you need a banded from a bandit like you just got bit in between the femoral, I got you charging up at the tip of the electro rod. Mine is not working right because of current signal strength at the thorax, not reflecting 7 up top and sending weak signals to the lower body, not enough to operate the pipe and ball.

They are many areas of the human body where you can find decay or buildup of dead muscle tissues. These obstructions are caused by miss-rotation of joints in the body from walking the wrong way; they are neither arthritis nor torn cartilage. The small toe is completely twisted and attaches itself to the ring toe, causing a deviation that locks the ankle from normal operation and also causing the placement of the fibula to be defective. During normal operation, the small toe and ring toe do work together, but they are not dependent on the movements of the big toe. The big toe, not receiving enough weight transfer; become jammed, causing the complete malfunction at the ankle, disabling the pump function of the heels and also causes a small deviation of the Tibia. The Tibia affects the knee as the Fibula affects the hips. The hips affect all of our organs as do the shoulders.

The feet have a 6 to 4 input and 2 to 3 output electrical conversion wire format, -2+1.

The right big toe is one negative working, as ground with the next two toes, as shock absorber and trigger to the tibia; the motion is descending. Ground is equal to 3.

The left small toe together with the ring toe, are one positive working with the next two toes as input lines to the fibula, by ways of the heel; the motion is in ascending order.

The 10 signals ignited from the ground, when the spring system is working, is 1 foot rotation added up before the heels resembling to the sacral with 1 charge. The feet focuses 12 signals into 10, the other 2 are used by the arms. There is a 13th signal which is ground and is only seen by the right big toe.

The coccyx is used only for energy transfer to and from the hips. When a signal 4 level 1 is transferred from the hips to the coccyx already at 4; that signal is transferred to the sacral, it becomes a stronger 4. The signal is amplified by repetition at the sacral when there's hip transfer, until it is strong enough to resemble a 5 alike the lumbar. The 5 lumbar does the same thing to remind the bottom of the thorax. Amplification happens when that signal strength 5 is meeting the erasable 7 coming from the cervical spine at the thorax. If the coccyx is not receiving a 4 signal from hip transfer; amplification cannot reach a true level 12 and the body slowly forgets its signature (regenerative capabilities), and gets old. The feet are almost a true mirror of the brain at 12 minus 2; the hands at 2 have a greater control over the cervical spine, the upper thorax and the primary electrical system.

These electrical signals that I am talking to you about do not activate the pelvic and make this process happen unless the heels are able to spring up and down. Walking on the heels as we do today, except for myself; the so called specialists do not have a record of what I'm talking about to compare. Bio-mechanical laboratories are scratching their heads right now. When the brain is able to use the feet as ground, the energy transfer is able to multiply itself up and down the spinal cord through pelvic magnetic friction. When someone walks on their heels, the signals do not have a clear ground. The heels being used as ground would not be logical in an electrical plant schematic; because of position and format. Not having a ground heats up the wires until some of them burn, lump and break. The brain eliminates electrical conduction completely in the lower body. That's when you can't dunk no more, stop having sidekicks and start thinking about retirement plans. The doctor's complaints are knee pain, back pain, neck pain, headaches, etc. O, same as you; he don't know that much. When three connections have breaks in their electrical wires, as it feels for an unused arm and two feet, the heart may not have enough room to pump and release "Oh, Oh, Santa bye-bye" (The Grinch).

The signal at the tail end of the spinal column should be a 5 at the sacral and a 4 at the coccyx. When people walk on their heels, after a certain age, the coccyx will not have a known usage or electrical signature in the spinal column. The sacral can't multiply the tail end with the signal 12 coming from the brain. The sacral becomes a 4. The lumbar will not accept it. The lower body becomes useless, hip problems, back problems, etc. At a young age, the coccyx will have conduction; the sacral is tightly placed but slightly moveable, with an electrical signature 4 at the coccyx resembling to the tail end of the signature 12 signal coming from the brain to the spinal column. Take a sit and be quiet, see I did not say that other word; I don't want to be rude, so silence! Listen, read, register, add, subtract, test and act. I'm the only specialist here! I'm a bush doctor, no paper degree; this is all hands on experience. This is indigenous medicine baby! The feet hit the ground, the veins and arteries contract, the hip balls activate the pelvic, the clavicles expand the sternum, I just bounced the ball, took one step, and dunked it in his face; did you see that, replay, replay please!

The breaks and accelerator are the nerves. The head and spine is not the support of the human body at all. Neither is the sacral the back wall of the hips. That doesn't even make sense, looking at the skeleton from the coccyx to C7, up to the brain. The coccyx is made to move inversely to the spinal column. It takes the hip casing and the clip of the ribs by the clavicles, to house the spinal column and relieve weight pressure on the sensitive nuclear reactor that God created, the brain!

The spring system, that is activated when the heels are free to move up and down, creates a signal that is amplified, and used to remind the brain of the signature 12 that is implanted within. The malfunction of the pump at the ankle is the beginning cause of all diseases co-parented by lack of perfusion, and half of the reason for failure of all organs. The pump function of the heels have an electrical pulse that is a major exciter of hip function and transfer of energy to the coccyx. Once the hurt is done at feet it is impossible to fix any other part of the body completely.

The tibia pulls on the fibula tearing it up so bad that doctors call it high ankle. There shouldn't be any breaks, bends or friction in that area. The exterior of the fibula where it's being pushed by the tibia is the second big circulation problem; the first is at the back of the heels. The deformation of the foot and the twist at the high ankle, as it's being called, are all caused by walking the wrong way, stepping with the heels first, adding descending and horizontal weight to the heels, where that area has the ability to float and works with vertical and ascending energy flow. Where are the mechanical engineers; is that type of design stable on its heels, would the spring motion operate if it were to land on its heels? Don't you have some robots with feet like that, how do they walk?

The heel has an electrical format of minus 2 ascending and plus 1 descending just like the feet. The 4 signals above the ankles below the knee cap resemble the sacral with one transfer from the coccyx. The heels have direct pull on R8 and may cause serious electrical overload to the heart and head when they are injured.

The knee caps act as the second magnifying balls of the human body from the ground up. We can say thank God for the knee cap. Its electrical format is -1+1 energy transfer down and up. Because of that ability to transform the two signals into one working signal for the femur to the hips; the knee caps make up for a great portion of the miss-fires from the heels and feet. However the array of wiring which covers the knee gets deteriorated as it tries to compensate for the twist coming from down under. The signals above the knee are the strongest 4 that is a 2 that is a 9 at the sacral at level 2. The knee cap passing freely around the meniscus is in direct proportion with the big toe's ability to detach itself from the heels.

They are two balls that attach the femur to the hips. In most human being, the left hip ball is stock at the Iliac and the right hip ball is too loose. If your scenario is as such as the previous sentence, than it's guaranteed that there will be a twist in your spine. When the hip is working, it transfers or receive 1/1 exact 4 energy transfer from symphysis pubis, to the coccyx, to the sacral. The capacity 12 signal harvested by the feet when they are walking on the toes, is concentrated into 10 signals before the heels, 4 before the knees, 2 before the hips, multiplied by 2 by hip transfer, magnetized in by the 4 vibrating at the coccyx. That signal can only reach capacity 12 again if there is hip transfer, in order to go through multiplication in the thoracic spine. The body works on the signature 12 that is in the brain; when someone walks on their heels, the hips don't pop to create friction, the brain is unfed with no amplification at the sacral, and it eats itself until death. The hips usually become defective, long after the ankles and knees have had problems. The hips are in relation with the ability of R8-7 to interact with the Xiphoid and the free-lance of the ankle and toes. The Xiphoid and the primary electrical system rarely support the demands of the brain and the heart for more than 100 years.

The shoulders and arms are in the primary electrical system of the human body. They are positive nodes only and cannot be used as ground by the brain and spinal cord. Only the feet can be used as such. The hands are great transmitters and partial receivers. The arms cannot activate the spring system. You must massage the shoulders and arms from the fingers to the sternum, and to the spinal column. After the hips are balanced, you'll be able to re-align all the joints and muscles deformed during the time you were walking on your heels; if you can take the pain. R1 through R7 are controlled by the scapula. The elbow, the thumb, the deltoid, the trapezoid and the breast must be re-aligned to fix the shoulder.

All of the vertebras belonging to the thorax can be physically controlled by the clavicles and a rib, but T8-12, associated with the Lumbar and the Sacral have a bigger impact on the spinal column overall. Anything wrong with the thorax then has an exact reflection at the sternum. The ribs slide close to each other and move in a circular motion, or bend with the spinal column and sternum; which makes it hard to detect its deformations. The spinal column bends and works in a circular motion as the hips and ribs do also. Its circular motion is dependent on the placement of the hips, T8 and the steering ability of the clavicles. Problems in the spinal column affect every single part of our lives.

There's no small spinal injury! Doctors rated my injury at 20%; I hate to see someone with 30% disability, as much pain as I have had to endure.

I'm at the head! I'm trying to trace for you a picture of the trajectory of the spring line within the skeleton. The first and most fined tuned 7 vertebras from the cervical spine serve as specialty signals for the 7 holes in our face. All parts of the body have a signature signal in the brain that is reflected to the spinal column. It's kind of hard to fix the head! There's at least going to be the possibility of bad thoughts. The skull contains the exact condition of the brain. By pushing the cerebellum and the face, the bones of the head can also be repositioned

When standing; all our body weight is transferred to the sternum by ways of R7-8. The clavicles have complete control of R1. Flow of electricity and speed of messages, are reliant on the positioning of the cervical ribs (the two ribs associated with the vertebra touching C7, so the two ribs connected to T1 (first thoracic vertebra), dissipated through R8-7; than to the parts at the bottom and front side of the rib cage, and sent back and forth and around to the spinal column by ways of the thoracic ribs. The clavicles are able to move the upper body around the spine without involving the hips; slightly twisting the lumbar.

The sternum is a spongy bone housing the 7 ribs coming from the top of the thorax. It is the master compensator and stabilizer of electricity in the body; using R1 as an overlap resistor. The sternum has the ability to break at R3 to create a different electrical path without affecting the heart or C7.

Because we're taking money from education and not teaching our kids to walk the right way; we are paying the price for many heart problems physical and mental disabilities, because a shoulder muscle is pulling a rib off the sternum. Many strokes and heart attacks can be attributed to the shoulder blades pulling on the cervical spine, causing a blockage of circulation to the head and the heart.

The information process goes into the stomach and inside the umbilical cord; there the final works are mirrored to transform energy signals to working electrical pulses able to operate our organs. The stomach muscles work as a unit with the clavicle and the Pubic, to maintain or fix the positioning of the sternum and the spine. The muscles of the stomach are made of a material that can always be manipulated back in place after any infractions in its position. The stomach is also the end point of the skin. I believe that all signals sent to the body have a corresponding ground at the umbilical. When reflective signals coming from defective feet are not true reflections of the output of the heart and the brain; symphisis pubis is de-harmonized gradually, and youth is lost.

The skin has a way to compensate for imperfection that I do not yet comprehend fully; but where ever something is wrong the skin gets pulled by it, and it hardens so the joint has a surface where it can be pulled. The hardening of the muscle ensures that electricity does not take that route; this will also limit movement. The skin acts as its own entity, and as the envelope of the human body.

The diaphragms work only when the human body is healthy, hips and shoulders in place, and energy transfer able to reach capacity 12.

Now that we have gone from the small toe through the heels favoring the fibula, up through the knee cap, to the hip and between the ribs and the spinal column, pass the neck, through the head, to both side of the face, to the shin, down the throat to the clavicle, to the sternum to the stomach and the skin. Now that we know that every single part of our body is affected from walking the wrong way. The big question is how to fix it? Education. Education. Education! When walking or running, the steps start on the toes, use both hands equally.

Sadly my worst adversaries in the battle to make this hypothesis a theory are intellectuals; specially the ones who learnt and do everything by the book, from ivy league universities, and somewhat are deaf to voices that may compromise their authority and cash flow. Sickness is a big business! I'm talking about people pretending to know it all, who can't run a mile, but would bolt for a roach. Yeah those sick doctors, liars, those kinds of pastors have made the road hard for anyone outside of their book awareness, to introduce any new ideas, and ask heavy questions in front of congress. Sir, Doctor General, is it true that there is a common defect in the human body after a certain age? Can that defect be prevented or fixed, and how? If the Doctor General is under oath, he better answer yes for the first part of the question. The second part, I'm the only one on Earth who can answer and demonstrate all its parts fully. So far what the specialists of the world have offered to you are pills, more sickness, high health care bills and no relief; except for some junkies I guess, who like to be high on prescription drugs. It is possible to completely stretch the body into comfort. The body must be operating on the spring line, which is only active while landing with the toes. During the sprint mode, the body does push and glide starting with the big toe, but that's not the motion that heals the body. The reception of the level 12 signal that could become a 4 at the coccyx after hip transfer is received while landing and starting the steps at the small toe and ring toe extremity.

Running is indispensable, when walking or running, the steps start with the ring toe, use both sides equally, both arms. There is no health without running. I know many advisers may have scared you away with bad knees and shin splints stories; but there is no way around the pain. If you are walking and running with the toes first, than all the pain you will feel, is a part of the body that was affected by accidents or by walking the wrong way moving back to its respective place. While running, learning how to land is the most important goal. You must lift the heels and the knees, for the feet to be able to land in a straight line, with the small toe and ring toe leading to the heels, and up the big toe. That process takes years to actually manifest the spring motion that starts at the foot. While counting 1, 2, 3, and breathe, keep your head up, shoulders up, knees up, heels up. Though it may sound easy on paper, I'm trying to tell you everything I know because it's so hard to gain health. The only way the pump at the heel works properly, is that the small toe and ring toe are free from any descending movements from the tibia. It took years of pounding and manually readjusting, before my feet started to land the right way, for me to feel how the spring pump works; this magnificent godly creation.

Only after the heels are able to move up and down can the hip balls be moved to allow maximum shock to the hips, for the amplification phase between the sacrum and the symphysis pubis to happen, by way of the coccyx. You don't need to run marathons nor 4 minute miles; but all that is possible if you start slow and build up to six miles. The most important gain in running is to rebalance each side equally the same, with the 1, 2, 3, motion, which shifts the body from the left to the right side. They are some pain to run with, and they are some other soreness to rest on. You should be your own trainer and teacher, only you can feel under your skin. We can talk and communicate; but it's up to you to put in application the parts you want to make your own. You can run for one hour or less; each time just try to stay in a straight line to fine health.

Stretching should be all the time, if only you knew how bad your body was twisted you would. They are so many ways you have to stretch; I will brush on a few. If you run and don't stretch before and after, you are defeating the purpose of the run; which is to shake and heat up the joints to be stretched. Once again you must listen to your body. They are many known stretching positions of healthy bodies, some of my favorites are; inside the wound sit down stand, Buddha bless you sit down stand, high fifth Jesus Christ cross stand, and the lion fist shaolin stand. I've done a lot of squats, lots of leg lifts, lots of sit ups, lots of shadow boxing and also stretching with weights. I'm still slow going back to doing pushups and swim the 50.I always try to run a fast pace 100 meter dash during my cross country runs.

Walking starting with the toes, flawlessly like a butterfly on a straight line, left foot first is actually harder while walking than running. There's even a stage that is so tricky, someone unsure like a child would keep on walking on the heels. They are many times that you may have to stump the ground with your heels, or stretch back on them; but it is illogical to habitually walk with the heels touching the floor first. It's as good to take slow walks, as it is to take fast ones. Go slow to be able to feel the toes grasping the ground like when walking down a steep hill, to feel the rotation pop the heels and lift up the side of the big toe. You can also walk fast to warm up the hips and the knees. The lion fist/Shadow boxing is my daily way to stretch. That's a quick 30 minute workout, starting with the stages of femininity (the serpent), to the rabbit, to the lion fist and kicks. I like shadow boxing because you can extend yourself fully without getting hit. With shadow boxing, you can safely train on both sides; the hook and upper cut are extremely important to loosen the shoulders. The kicks help to stretch the hips. Dancing to music helps the body to float like in sexual intercourse. Have you ever tried to do these movements without music or a partner? I know that sex and rock and roll were forbidden subjects back in the days, but it's actually healthy to dance and mate. The feeling of pre-climax gives us an extra strength we are unable to achieve without. The body is able to generate enough energy to spasm, which is needed to align back ribs.

Playing a sport has some spiritual attributes that are the third party that makes getting healthy mystical. But wait there's more! You will get hurt if you're playing hard. Would you think that a twisted ankle is actually good, or would you call a dislocated hip lucky? The ankle, the hips, the shoulders are three fail safe joints! Thank you God I said, now I just need to fix the other side.

I wanted to play in the NBA, I still think of myself as the best guard ever. Now it has become more WNBA, the way the refs are calling those girly technical fouls, just for looking at the subject of your new website post; so I'm going to get back to basketball, we must start at the first basic sport which is football. Still the most popular sport in the world, the original football teaches the kick that resemble the signal sent by the heels when operating properly in the body. It's good to teach children that sport first also because at young ages they forget quickly and can't remember or register you've told them not to walk with the heels first; but also at a young age, if they are reminded and educated; they retain and apply information better than any adult learner. The header is only found in football, and is why I'm able to heal my body even after so many injuries. The header stretches the body in a way that creates a computerized signal that goes through the body to fix the spring line, and that signal can always be reactivated by the header movement. You can feel the joints pulling all the way down to the toes when executing the header, just juggling the ball one on one, for technical practice.

The second sport that I wish to brush on is American football. I've seen some roughing the passer calls that are shady, in the name of football players. But American football, just like Hockey; still remain a game for gladiators. You know boys will be boys, sometimes we fight eh! I love American football, not just because I like to see a receiver get flipped in the air, fall down, and don't move. I also enjoy seeing a quarterback, on his quarterback after he got blindsided, side-lined, carried out by four men waving with two fingers on a golf cart. Come on, you know if you're a real safety you're trying to knock somebody out, cold, hit the road Jack, don't you come back no more. You want to see it happen to opposite team only, if you're a real football junky; that's fair enough play! I don't believe they penalized some players for bounty hunting. Dog! Every player in the NFL knows this could be their last play. Dude! You've got three seconds to get rid of the ball;

or else that's your balls. I mean testicles this time. Anyway, take it how you want it. I'm getting carried away. Yeah! I'm a bad ass nigger! American football provides the basic four, three, two point positions, to help the body ball down to the ground. The play sets, during a goal line running play, would show you best how low everyone is, and how you should try to stretch. The four and three point positions allow the head or the hips to pull at T1 and T12 in the thoracic spine. The thoracic spine is the most flexible part of the spinal column.

As much as they respected each other as great players, it was war on the court between Magic and Bird. Oakley was saying to Michael, I will hit you every time you come in here. Sir Charles was booty banging the whole NBA off the paint. Shawn Kemp was pre-writing the script for the Matrix. Isaiah was dribbling, passing and shooting them down! The fly by, by Worthy look like today's 3-D video games! The Dikembe none of that; the trash talks and response back! The crowd booing a free throw shooter! Basketball is to me the best sport to exemplify a complete sport to provide good health. The love of basketball has been my second helper. My dreams to be like Mike had made me relentless. I must get there or bust. Bust! Something inside my body was stopping me more than ever! But nothing can stop me, as I know that one day, if I keep on running and walking the right way with my toes first, I will be healthy and I will play. I am still mastering my dribble and my shot, but most of all I'm trying to fix my steps. I've got your OG right here son! Come get some! I have gained enough confidence in my hypothesis to write this book; I can take you and you to the rim. You can't guard me solo or that's 2 and one, as your reaction was to slow.

I will, I can, and I must manually, forcefully fix every single inch of my body. Beside the walking, the running and stretching; you must know the physiology of the human body also to finalize its healing. Most of my injuries became a starting point to compare against the other side. When a joint dislocates, it falls to its lowest point. The skeleton is on its way down, might as well help it. Don't you see, you get shorter as you get older anyway?

When an effort or movement had made my body turn across the joints of T1 to T7; the pain would tear me down to tears and desolate pasture. I noticed a black nail on the left ring toe. The ankle, knee and hip felt completely un-wheeling on the left side; shoulder and ribs including. There was a bulge in the middle on the left side of the Thorax that my body was trying to avoid. That's what we're going to do next; we're going to pull the skin down from the toes to the head.

1. With one hand under and one over, thumbs between the ring toe and middle toe, maneuver up to the ankle joint, take left thumb to small toe ball, go down small toe and back up between small toe and ring toe to small toe ball. Keep left thumb with pressure there.

2. Take right thumb across the ankle joint to the big toe line all the way to the bottom of the big toe and the index, or pointing finger toe. Take left thumb and also bring that line

back around under. Take both middle fingers to meet at toe joint 2 and 4 counting the spacing from the small toe.

3. Take both middle fingers and slide under foot to meet as a triangle at the tip of the heel. Make another triangle up to the top of the heel behind the foot, at the connection of the posterior Tibial. Bring the triangle back down across tibia and heel and fibula and heel to joint where the ankle meets the foot across top and straight line down across top of toes 3 and 4.

4. With thumbs on each side of the posterior Tibial, put other fingers between tibia and fibula and roll fibula away from that spot they're calling high ankle; because it's broke, an han! The tear and deformation at that area is caused by pushing wrongly on the heels. The tibia, the fibula, the femur, the hip must sit on a spring. This type of structure is not so strong and stable standing straight on its heels. When walking or running the steps start with the toes. Look at the picture; the foot is a mechanical spring, amazing when you learn to use it.

5. Bring the fingers up; there's a clear path all the way up to the outside of the knee joint. Take left hand to exterior side of the knee touching the fibula. Take right hand across front, between knee cap and tibia, to the anterior side of the knee touching the tibia. Work a lot on those two spot with middle and ring finger.

6. Take thumbs to the middle top of knee cap at the connection with the femoral. Pull skin down at the bottom of knee cap. In a circular motion, go deep and repair the connection at the popliteal. Take the two middle fingers back down pulling the tibia away from the fibula this time. On the way up we were pulling more on the fibula away from the tibia.

7. Take both thumbs and hands, push down on the connection of the left Femoral with the Pubic. Push on the left side of the Pubic in a down motion, as if trying to meet the two thumbs pushing left, to defuse the connection.

8. Take both thumbs to the top of the left iliac crest and pushes down and left. Pull right hip ball up.

9. Take both middle fingers to meet at the connection of the sacral and the lumbar. Pull the skin down to retrieve it from the coccyx. The skin twisted at the top of the Anus is the cause of Prostate cancer in men. This line cannot be untwisted without softening its electrical circle.

10. Go back up the spine with thumbs on each side of the spinal column and out at R12. The floating ribs, as modern medicine are the bottom poles of the circular motion and control the bending ability of the human body. These ribs work together as the bottom shaft of the clavicles and the hips. R7-8 are the top.

11. Work towards the front of the body takes the thumbs up to meet at the tip of the sternum. Pull everything down as you go up towards the clavicle. Push left and down on R7 and R1.

12. Take both hands and forcefully pull ribs to take equal parts off the sternum. Move R1 from under the clavicle.

13. Also work at unwinding the ribs from the spinal column, by pulling on the Latissimus Dorsi, up to the trapezius out to the deltoid at the tip of your shoulder blades. The trapezius is out of alignment with its connection at C7 and T1; you know that spot where you feel the bad neck ache. There also the deltoid is pulling on the trapezius so badly that it causes a bulge. This line is also premature and would have disappeared if a person was taught to use that arm alike the other.

14. it's guaranteed to have an imbalance at the shoulders, if there is an imbalance at the hips that causes the joint of L1 and T12 to tilt even a micro-inch on any side. The joint at T12 and L1 is like a ball inside a hole within the spinal column.

15. You must pull on the deltoid as to twist the arm inward to forcefully re-separate the muscles. Hold the triceps on both side of the elbow, going down across the radius to the ulna, bring thumb around for middle finger and thumb to meet at radius. Work hand down to

wrist with thumb on the palmar arches and fingers on carpals.

16. Work on fingers like toes. Nails and hair are a good looking type of wax and boogie, or fetus. There I said it. Nice looking hair girlfriend. The circular motion to work on the hands is as separating the muscles between the wrist and the thumb.

17. Take middle fingers and place them on the thorax, pull down towards the cervical spine; work on connection of the jugular vein behind the ear. Across to the temporal bone to the top of the eye structure, down to the nose and around the eye sockets to the bottom of the ear, down the jugular vein to the clavicle.

18. The clavicles, working together with a tight stomach, are able to move ribs with the thorax; without moving the hips or the head. This capability helps to fix the alignment of the ribs between the sternum and the thorax.

19. Massage vigorously the connection between the clavicle and the sternum pushing everything in a downwards motion again.

20. Take hands to both side of the thorax and slide down with pressure towards the sacral, out the balls of the hip and do it all over again a million times until the body is moving freely.

The head is the top 2 circles at the top of the conductive rod; the arms and legs make up the other 2 circles which can be divided into 4. The occipital bone is the Sacral of the head; providing support and stability to the spinal column at the entrance of the head. C7 is solid, C1 is suspending.

The frontal bone belongs to the face and is barely mobile like the occipital bone. The temporal bone is extremely mobile.

Down to the jaw bone to the area where the wisdom teeth gave man wisdom, like my spinal injury had forced me to learn the human body.

With the hips and shoulder being out of place; I'm surprised there aren't more strokes and heart diseases in our statistics. What is the main cause of death in the world? Heart disease! Check out the pectoralis being pulled by the deltoid at R3! Some of these connections once again are premature. They were supposed to go away like the other side that you are able to throw with. Have you tried to write or pitch with the weak side? You wouldn't dare use a knife with your none-writing hand, have you ask yourself why?

A coma is a state of unconsciousness, where the brain is not dead but it's unable to order the body. A coma can be reversed with repositioning or exciting the body. C7 has to be affected either by C1 ,T1 , T3, T8 or L5 for physical interaction with the brain to stop, or there must be a head injury.

During a cervical spine fracture, a ring will come off C1 and affect the throat and C6. In a Thoracic fracture; a ring will come off T1 and affect the scapula and T8. A Lumbar tic fracture will affect T12 and L5. For a head injury Coma; the bone involve must have crossed the grey matter area, and it will affect the face. The temple, the cheeks and the jaw bones, along with the eyes, the nose and the frontal lobe as a fixe can be used to displace any injuries to the head. By kneeling and leaning patient backwards and twisting the shoulders back and forth; the electrical system of the human body can almost always be restarted.

In extreme cases with unknown injuries; the left ring toe, the right thumb, the right big toe, the left ring toe must be injured. The right middle quadrant and the left lower quadrants must be punctured 1in and 1/2in respectfully. The Anus wall can also be broken to push the electrical lines. The idea with the cause of coma is unknown is to transfer the pain to a workable location by the brain.

In a coma caused by the spinal column; R8 must be re-aligned to free the Xiphoid by pulling down on the chest cavity. The relationship between R1, the scapula and R8 is almost always repairable by untwisting the Vena Cava. Although Oxygen is helpful during Coma, banging on the chest is not; twisting the body left, right, back and forth is more practical in restarting an electrical system. The application of an AED should have its positive wire at the left ring toe and negative at right big toe.

The toes will only stretch through walking and running as you start the steps with them. The heels will pop; the ankles and hip will start to move up and down, the circular motion will be regained around R8. The clavicle will be able to steer the skin and muscles to the tip of the toes. The muscle and joint pain will diminish slowly, the headaches too; as the spine becomes freer. This pain feels so good, knowing that it's going away!

When the head bends, the pressure is felt at the top of T1 and R1 across the sternum. When the whole upper body bends, the pressure is felt at the bottom of L5and at R7 up front.

A hip imbalance where the pelvic girdle crosses the right line is felt on the left side of the Iliac. A hip dislocation affects the lumbar and the reproductive organs.

The lines from the scapula, wrongly connected to the spinal column, along with a rock solid ankle (glued together), are the cause of imbalance at the hips and spinal column.

In most of our lives there's ankle, knee, hip, back and neck problems; not counting the headaches and other vermin eating away at our hopes and dreams. These oinks will not go away through magic; they must be attended to with great perseverance. The brain and the heart do not have handles to hold and twist and fix. We must begin with the physical terminals, the meat and bones, to unify the human body, mind and soul.

All muscular and joint pain is due to the irregular rotation of the body from walking the wrong way. When walking or running, the steps start on the toes. There is no health without running. You must count 1, 2, and 3 in your head as you walk and run in a straight line. Heels up, knees up, head up, shoulders up, breathe. I can still feel my shoulder blades friction against the rib cage; it needs some more work and adjustment. Now that my hips are still almost re-aligned and my ankles almost loose, I am almost sure when I stand in front of the doctors of the world to tell them: stop that train! The foot having lost its elasticity is at the base of all our aches and pain! When walking or running, the steps start with the toes. Let's correct our problem. Let's legalize marijuana worldwide. Let's have a party on Earth. This time it's going to be forever in the name of God.

This ancient practical way to heal the human body called Acupressure extended more than just to fix the body by walking and running on the toes; it was aimed at enhancing the ability of the mind to expand its vision, way beyond Physics and Chemistry.

Knowledge is power. With so many outrageous spirits, the selfish has molded information and bended the truth, with personal feelings to control population with corporation.

Teachers build leaders not slaves; Pharaohs are always reborn to revolt. The attempt to domesticate a human is to dig a hole, and wait because you will fall in it.

Breathing, aligning the Pubic and walking are things that we can best do for ourselves; they are also indispensible to our health. We must give the future a chance. Teach the children how to walk starting their steps on the toes. Show them through good examples how to work on themselves. Education is not a privilege, it's an obligation!

The Big Toe!

There is no health without running! When walking or running the steps should start on the toes. Notice a child learning how to walk. Before the age of three, they proceed to walk on their heels. At that young age, it is impossible for a child to know; that the pain is part of the payment for the gift of life. When we jump rope, going down the stairs, landing from a dunk; we never do these things on the heels; that are because there is no elasticity to absorb any shock falling that way. Until the big toe has the proper bend; the rest of the body has no chance to work properly.

After too many years walking on my heels, every other joint was affected. The lining that controls the joint is what needs to be manually, forcefully pushed back and twisted into its place. There is no torn cartilage to be cut out. In my opinion, it is illogical to cut a muscle unless in case of an emergency.

All muscular and joint pain is due to the improper rotation of the body, from walking the wrong way. Most defective organs are due to hypo-perfusion; whether it is from lack of oxygenated blood, or irregular electrical pulses.

The heels block the passage to the toes, the pain is felt at the ankles, knees, hips and spine. The bones crack and squeak, from the imbalance of the left to the right side of the body. When the muscles are no longer able to give and compensate, they tear apart, or they dislocate a joint.

With our known health system, when someone reaches the age of forty, he or she is considered old, done, retired; their body has been defeated. It surprises me, that elite professional athlete, would get operated on, by doctors whom have never made it. The doctor can't run a mile, how can he fix a knee that is wrong in his body? You are the best doctor for yourself.

My friends know thyself; stop complaining about every little pain; learn how to make your movements perfect. Health is your wealth. No one can walk for you; you must learn to land these steps on the road.

I have never seen a dead man walk or talk. Why are you waiting for death to find life? Eternal life is through life. Life is not cheap and you can't buy it. You have to work on yourself every day of the week. Walk right! A woman gives life! The steps are feminine. O, well! When walking or running, the steps start on the toes.

Written by God!

God is made of all the different seven colors of the rainbow. God is great, God must be mad. To each side of the story there is an opposition. No matter how righteous or how insane something may seem; someone somewhere think that it is normal or abnormal.

Now I'm wondering inside my head; what is right or wrong, what is good or bad; does it matter? We spend all our lives fighting for or against something, to find out after years of inner battle that we have very little say, and our influence really will not make the world turn this way or that way, not even one inch.

I thought we were civilized, and gone away from the ways of savages. I am slowly realizing that most of the answers are biased in many ways. If I am wrong than God, he is wrong; but cultural rights and self- oriented ideas should be eliminated from the skies of thoughts, surely they should not override human rights, and Godly ways.

No one should be forced to enter a cult of bloodshed, where their ability to love and their souls will be taken away. Insanity has nothing to do with God and the logic behind laws and commandments, which could be said to have been written with the help of the Holy Spirit and so, by the hands of God.

Be God. Follow no one. We all have been influenced. There's a war inside of me. I must find peace, Inner peace. They'll never be justice. God is multicolor. I took a side. The righteous suffers. I accept the pain to love. Some words are wisdom, and can be said to be words of God, written by God.

Mind programming!

They think of themselves as descendants of an animal. Good lord. Now look how man living alike a cannibal. With no care, nor honor for its prey; he goes around and devours all who dare to stand in his way. Tattooed up to the neck he belongs to the click. It's a closed dark circled only get in if you know exactly where you fit. For the money man will steal, bleed and kill. Now he's wealthy with material to show, just how vain he is. To justify mass murdering they'll called my people savages. We had agricultural tools; they had gun powder, cannon balls and bullets. But their mind is programmed.

Thousands of containers loaded with food on the dock; each with an expiration date. Every day the boss decides which ten trailers he will destroy, to make room for new fresher goods. The security guard has his orders to stop anyone attempting to dumpster dive for the still good fruits and vegetables. They are children hungry that could use the expired yams and potatoes. I thought we were civilized people where we take care of each other. It took me a long time, but now I see we're still living in a dog eat dog man eat man society. When a Roman breaks the law it's a mistake, when it's someone else it's a crime. Our mind is programmed.

HEALTH IS!

The Ivy League or World Health Organization declares that" Health is the complete physical, mental, and social well-being, and not merely the absence of disease or infirmity. "As I was reading further in the documents written by the WHO, this definition is mostly oriented towards mental health, and it further confirms my own analogy of world governments in its entirety. Our leaders are a whole bunch of sick drunks with an intellectual degree; they have a specific group of people they intend to include or exclude in their definition of health. Just like capitalistic democracy is a system tailored to fit only a few; the description of Health given by the World Health organization is written so apartheid can be justified. Physical and mental health does work hand in hand; but the emphasis should be a lot more on the body first, than the mind.

I remember one day I decided to keep on playing ball, knowing that my mother would come back from work to find me outside dirty and sweaty, and with my school obligations undone. The consequence was a rage oriented leather belt to my thighs, and a century in the corner on my knees it seems. My dreams of following Dr.J to the NBA had to take a back seat, second to my lawyer mom's dedication to direct me towards law or medicine; the only professions valuable in her book. I wanted to focus on physical health, hang out with the thugs, and master ball handling. She wanted me to get an A in French literature, wear my white Pierre Cardin shirt and Christian Dior tie; and sit in the court room; to brush shoulders with her colleagues.

I’ve always had a problem with ireliable authorities. The WHO states that; “There is no health without mental health." When you have a headache, or a tooth ache, is your mind healthy? The brain only works properly when there is no obstruction in its oxygen, nutrients and electrical supply. The body cannot be an adequate conductor when the signals cannot reach the ground because of obstruction towards or at the feet. The organs deteriorate faster when there is misconduct ion of electricity within the body. There is no health without running. When walking or running, the steps should start on the toes.

Now days, everyone is talking about healthy food. I've had to inform my daughter's instructor that I am a runner and an X-boxer, and that they are healthy habits; no such thing as healthy food. There can be GMO, which are bad for you; but our body is able to metabolize almost everything and use it.

If we were to mathematically analyze the definition of health written by our so called leaders; our computation would start with: Health is the complete physical well-being, but none of these intellectuals can run the 100 meter dash under 11 seconds, nor play basketball with college kids at 48; so they bypass the beginning which is the most important part.

How does life start on Earth for the human kind? Everyone crawls and start to gain balance on their toes! The original sin is, all of us will take one bad step, and all of us will than start walking on our heels. The brain will be less capable because of the body being affected by the imbalances in its original structure. It's than impossible for the mind to function completely with all its capability without physical health.

The teaching that a person is left or right handed is also a major contribution in physical sickness. The muscles of the shoulder, on the weak side or the least used arm, become improperly attached to the rib cage, creating the majority of heart problems known to man today.

Ignorance kills more people than bullets; when it's our leaders teaching ignorance, than it's like a bomb. "Thirty minutes a day of physical exercise", is considered to be the minimum standard per the WHO! "Biking, walking and dancing" are recommended, but I saw nothing on running. What must happen to unlock the ankles, happens in the air; meaning that you must be running for it to happen.

It takes years, of pounding on the toes, before they retake their normal form, and for the mind to gain confidence landing on them. I read nothing on stretching in the WHO's documents, which also constitute a major part of physical health.

Life- saving skills.

The primary cause of death in America and around the world is heart diseases. Someone is holding the left side of their chest, breathing uncomfortably, than they just fall on the ground. What do you do? The first ten minutes after a heart attack is critical to the patient's survival rate, it is called the chain of survival. When you find a person on the ground, they are three steps you can quickly take to help save their lives.

Early activation of the Emergency Medical Services is required, than early CPR, and thirdly early application of an Automatic Exterior Defibrillator. Cardiopulmonary resuscitation is an extremely important lifesaving skill to learn. According to the American Heart Association, heart disease is contributing to 330,000 deaths per year in

America. The major heart problem reoccurring in adults is an irregular heartbeat rhythm due to electrical disturbance. If you suspect someone is having a heart - attack, the first thing to do is to activate the EMS system, Emergency Medical services can be reached by dialing 9-1-1. This number will automatically activate the Fire department, the Police and the Ambulances.

The ambulances most importantly in a medical emergency, will have advanced life support services which includes the administration of vital medications, the application of special breathing devices, they are also equipped with AED's to administer defibrillation shocks. When available, an AED, automatic external defibrillator is used primarily to treat heart attack patient.

When the heart has no electrical output, this condition of the heart is called ventricular fibrillation, it usually requires an electrical shock to jump start the heart back to a regular beat. There is a guideline to follow before applying an AED to a patient; the person must be unresponsive, breathless and the heart must have a ventricular fibrillation signal which is detected by the automatic exterior defibrillator.

In most cases however, the first responder does not have an AED than CPR becomes the second most important step and must be administered continuously to give the EMS system time to bring advanced life support to the scene. There is less risk for brain damage and the survival rate extends immensely when CPR is performed promptly.

When you approach someone you think is having a medical problem, you gently shake them; ask them if you could help them and if they are O.K. Put your ears close to their face and listen for breath sounds. If the person is still unresponsive, immediately dial 911 and begin CPR. Make sure they are not just taking a nap and that it looks like an accidental scenery.

To start CPR, you first need to clear the airway. You do that by tilting the victim's head back with one hand pushing on the forehead and the other pulling on the chin. After obtaining an airway, you give the victim 2 deep slow breath mouth to mouth while holding his nasal passage close and assuring a chest rise. Make sure you are in a comfortable position, because the next step may be strenuous. Begin the count for 30 chest compressions by placing the heel of one hand wrapped around the other, in the middle of the chess and pushing downwards about one inch at a "Staying Alive" rate. After each 30 compressions, give 2 breaths, and continue this cycle until EMS arrives.

According the American Heart Association, there are over 330,000 deaths per year caused by heart failure. The person who needs help might be a close relative in your home. You can save a life if you know these three simple steps. Activate the EMS system, call 911; obtain an airway by tilting the patients head back and pulling on the chin; begin CPR, 2 breaths per 30 compressions per minutes. Connect an AED to the patient as soon as possible, proceed for a rapid transport.

Getting my Red Cross rescuer CPR certification is one of my prized achievements. Don't fall out in front of me; you're not going to die on my watch.

Depression/ an emotional feeling!

The side effects of mistreatment are far worse than no treatment. The inability for doctors to say I don't know has caused them to wrongly medicate and incidentally create more harm than the existing symptoms.

Depression in most cases is the result of an event with negative ending. It can easily be deterred by changing or adding a different positive to the environment. It is not degradation in mental capability or a physical disability. It is the natural response of the body, mind and soul, and also it's the beauty of human nature to have such deep expression.

Though there may be chemical changes when someone is depressed, which is normal; I completely disagree with the classification of depression as a disease, it is an emotional feeling influenced by an outside force and cannot be measured.

I'm supposed to be the kid to fix this dysfunctional world; I've had this burden on my shoulders ever since I can remember. The weight of its difficulty has often questioned my faith and brought tears to my days. Are you kidding me? Fixing this world is impossible!

No, I think the people of Earth are just depressed! What is depression? It's an emotional disorder that has been extensively researched relating to feelings of hopelessness and despair!

Are you not a psychiatrist? Aren't there any good treatments for depression established already? What is your prescription? By changing the perception of success in someone's life, the mind leaves the low levels of self-esteem and sadness and climb out in an acceptable land of happiness. Yes, I'm an expert on the subject through life experience and I've also done some research. I do not agree with the present classification of depression as a disease.

According to the encyclopedia Britannica, "depression, in psychology, is a mood or emotional state that is marked by feelings of low self-worth or guilt and a reduced ability to enjoy life". But a more exclusive definition can be seen on the five o'clock city bus. As you looked in a depressed person's face; their lives are instantly aging before your eyes, their magnetism is openly uninviting, their conversation is vague, and their language is negative. As you approach a depressed person, your energy suddenly weakened, your mood becomes affected, and your own health can be immediately infected.

By telling you the story that has put them in a sad state, an emotional friend can sometimes make you cry, hug and kiss, smoke and drink alcohol together in misery. Sometimes depression can turn to anger and elevate mood swings to become bipolar disorder, and involve you in domestic violence.

They are many side effects of depression that we may be able to scientifically measure and more serious mental and physical health issues deriving from depression that may be curable through medication, but depression itself is an emotional feeling; man cannot cure emotions with chemicals.

Laura A King, Ph.D. the author of Science of Psychology defines depression as a mood disorder," Mood disorders are psychological disorder in which there is a primary disturbance of mood". They are many life experiments that can cause someone to be depressed. For example, everyone falls in love; weather it's with a person or a thing.

The loss of love is usually an immediate engine carrying depression. Someone whom has died in older ages seems to bring less pain than when it's a young one who's died. Sometimes two people are madly in love and one don't know the other is especially in love with the sex, and she gets emotionally shattered by the sudden emptiness in her heart when she finds out he's cheating. Job hunting and disappointment, not enough cash to fulfilled the higher expectations of life, unable to see a way out from a dark tunnel; all are attributes of the feeling, that develop from within, that we call depression.

I do not agree with MS King however for classifying depression as a hereditary trait; I would prefer that she stated the truth as far as being born in a depressive system in society, the majority of the population will be depressed.

Pharmaceutical drug therapy, shock treatment and psychotherapy are three types of treatment being utilized today for depressive disorder patients. They are many antidepressant agents being used in our medical world today. One well known medication on the modern medicine market today is Prozac. Which the active ingredient is supposedly intended to correct the chemical imbalance in the brain that causes depression. In the research "The utilization of antidepressants and Benzodiazepines among people with major depression in Canada"; it was found that the side effects of the drug, includes tolerance and dependency.

Though the research made so far indicates a brain activity that may be chemically challenged; emotions are attached to the beat of the heart so depression can only be cured by repairing the cause. Is it more intelligent to replace a normal reaction from the human body with a different environment, than to risk drug addiction, liver diseases and heart problems?

But instead of accepting that depression cannot be medically approached in all cases, doctors prefer to go deeper in the brain to search for clues, and they call it major depressive disorder. This is where we get the term medical practice.

Electric shock therapy is where an electrical wave is sent through someone's brain; which I think is like a bodily punishment to kids that parents really don't like; so they force them to be obedient and responsive by torture and fear, this type of therapy is usually used when the depressive behaviors have escalated into violent and bipolar disorders.

The most efficient form of therapy to really waste your time and money in my eyes is counseling. Marcia Clemmitt claims, “in recent decades, psychotherapy for depression made great strides, as research provided evidence that some “talk” therapies are effective especially cognitive behavioral therapy.“ She spent the whole hour taking about her own teen age daughter and their depressive relationship.

Depression is a 27 billion dollar business and it also feeds other research industries, especially drug abuse. Richard, L, Worsnop writes “In the United States alone, it is estimated that severe depression affects more than 15 million people. It is so widespread that it is sometimes called “the common cold of mental illness.”

My take on the subject include almost no respect to the present treatments for depression. The drug market is essentially trying to create a pill for every aspect of life. Failed expectations are always at the base of depression. The so call higher ups in charge are holding tight to the chain of financial stability. The wages are regulated so that someone in their forties will for sure to go to a midlife crisis.

Education that is available to the mass is so that you know enough to work for the owner, but never be able to breathe on your own, and never become self-sufficient.

Now days God and prayer is like synonymous to uncool, the stories of molestation of young boys in the church pool does not help the reputation of the clergy. These are the origin of the problem of depression, when there isn't order in our lives we become depressed. The parasite (controlling authority in this case) must be eliminated to cure depression.

Not having a depressed population would essentially create a revolution. Happy people usually want to smoke weed and drink beer while listening to music bathing in the sun all day at the beach; they don't want to work for minimum wage at the factory.

I do like the field of psychology, but is there a race to put a stamp on I created this, I did this, and I invented this! All while staying in the corporate boundaries; our doctors are making beaucoup cash medicating the poor ignorant.

Depression alike many other mental disorders tagged as diseases are in actuality results of everyday facts of life. I do agree with many scientists who don't believe emotions can be measured and therefore depression should not be classified as a disease.

Giving drugs to a young woman that has lost her husband to one of the bridesmaid is simply getting her high so she forgets him momentarily.

Paying the worker a descent amount so he could buy his own house and insurance and maybe have a little garden with a couple of goats in the back yard would solve his scary facial expression coming from his depression.

The archbishop should not be examining back pockets in the confession room; that subject is a depressive one. I feel as if a big scam in the health system is defining new sickness to treat and medicate.

Are we really healthier ten years after all these inventions? The American dream is to one day have a dog, a cat and a house, kids, friends and a pretty wife, a mustang and a boat, a shotgun and some hooks, maybe a few important books. When these things are not in place, it's easy to get depressed. Oh! I forgot about the Harley Davidson.

We have luxurious needs and Cinderella fairy tale dreams. A person does not need drug treatment and medicine for depression because he can't afford the brand new 2012 Alpha Romeo. Give him a lottery ticket, some weed, cigarettes and alcohol; this is just as good medicine as any of the prescribed drugs and treatments available in modern medicine. I say, if you are going to kill them anyway at least let them have a little fun and be happy for a few moments.

Only the powerful writers were allowed to write in the Bible, they were not necessarily disciples. They are many influential figures in the medical society and their stamp of approval may very well make believers out of a half blind society.

The introduction of high computer resolution is giving researchers a new look at activities in the brain. It is normal to have reactions in the brain from any types of feelings. Love and happiness, sadness and depression, all fall under the category of emotions. Some adolescents get love sick, I pray we don't start to give them hate pills to counter. Depression is a normal sensation of lost and disappointment. Depression is not a disease, but an emotional feeling.

Abortion and Crime!

Abortion is considered to be a crime by many and a woman's right of reproduction freedom by others. The Supreme Court defines viability to be after 24 weeks of pregnancy. Before the third trimester, abortion is legal in all states as a woman's right of privacy, between her and her physician. After 24 weeks, the law that governs abortion has certain restrictions before it is applied.

Is the legalization of abortion a major denominator in the decrease of other violent crimes? Though they are other situations besides the mother's health where an abortion could be logical; they do not to include the third trimester and should not be used as a mode of birth control. A healthy choice can only be made on a case by case basis when approaching a subject as sensitive as abortion.

Some researchers say that the five states that legalized abortion between 1968 and 1970 experienced an earlier drop in violent crime rate than states that legalized murder at a later date. Abortion was legalized state wide after the Roe verses Wade case on 22, Jan, 1973. Roe versus Wade is the class action suit of a woman against the laws of Texas allowing abortion only if a woman's health was in danger because of the pregnancy. Roe raised the possibility of unwanted birth and provided the court with examples where these types of pregnancies may be harmful regardless if they were directly related to a woman's health. The Judges, unable to suggest abstinence, found that Roe and her colleagues presented enough justifiable evidence to overturn the current laws. The ruling of the court was based on the fact that the laws in place violated the fourteenth and the ninth amendments which protects the constitutional rights of a woman to have an abortion.

The stage was set for an all- out war between women rights activists and anti-abortion groups. Each side was coming up with different strategies to support their own views. Many clinics have been burned, some bombed and many doctors have been killed or persecuted for supporting such law that allows the termination of an unborn child. Even at the State-level, though they are forbidden to ban abortion, they have made it as difficult as possible for a woman to get such service.

The decision to allow woman to legally obtain an abortion was opposed by many during the Roe versus Wade case, to include Harry Blackmun, William J. Brennan, Chief Justice Warren Burger, William O. Douglas, Thurgood Marshall, Lewis Powell and Potter Stewart. Some doctors claim that an unborn child is a fetus and is not considered as the beginning of life. Others think specifically during the third trimester, that the removable of an unborn child is partial birth. There have been many cases where a child being aborted is born alive and the doctors than have to kill that child to complete the abortion.

In an article written by Michael J New, “Using Natural Experiments to Analyze the Impact of State Legislation on the Incidence of Abortion. Heritage Foundation, Jan, 23, 2006, 15. www.heritage.org/Research/Family/cda06-01.cfm. He writes:

"Many medical experts disagree. The courts said the law is too broad, potentially applying not only to what some doctors call a "dilation and extraction" procedure (D&X) but also to the more commonly used abortion procedure: a "dilation and evacuation" (D&E).The law itself begins by graphically defining "partial-birth abortion" as a procedure in which a physician "vaginally delivers a living, unborn child's body" until "the entire head" or "any part of the baby's trunk past the navel" is outside the body and then kills the "partially delivered infant by an overt act (usually the puncturing of the back of the child's skull and removing the baby's brains)."

Kenneth Josh. Abortion debates: will more restrictions be enacted? Library.cqpress.com/CQ researcher. 2, March, 2003, Web, 15, April, 2011. He reports:

"The battle lines on the abortion issue remain clearly drawn 30 years after the Supreme Court's controversial Roe v. Wade decision established a constitutional right to the procedure during most of a pregnancy. Anti-abortion groups continue to urge Congress and state legislatures to regulate abortion practices, while abortion-rights supporters say the measures undercut a woman's reproductive freedom. At the urging of President Bush, Congress is moving to ban a late-stage procedure that opponents call "partial-birth" abortion, although the Supreme Court struck down similar state law years ago. "Although abortion is legal in every state, it is not necessarily available in every state. In Mississippi, for example, there is only one abortion clinic that services the entire state, and it only performs abortions up to 16 weeks.

One strategy used by the anti-abortion movement involves driving abortion clinics out of business, which arguably serves the same function as a state-level ban.

Kenneth Josh/Kathy Koch: Abortion Showdown: will the latest anti-abortion moves succeed? Library.cqpress.com/CQ researcher. 22, September, 2006, Web, 15, Apr, 2011.

South Dakota has become the latest battlefield in the abortion wars. A Nov. 7 referendum will let voters approve or reject a new law aimed at banning virtually all abortions in the state. South Dakota legislators passed the law earlier this year in a direct challenge to the Supreme Court's landmark 1973 decision, Roe v. Wade, which legalized abortion during most of a woman's pregnancy. Abortion -rights advocates in South Dakota forced a referendum on the measure, which would allow abortions only if necessary to protect a woman's life.

More disturbingly, to justify their insanity, a group of so called specialists and experts have even gone to the extent of promoting abortion by stating that its legalization has a direct impact on violent crimes being committed in our society.

Steven D. Levitt/ John J. Donohue III. The impact of legalized abortion on crime. Papers.ssrn.com. Quarterly journal of economics. May, 2001, Web, 15, April, 2011.

We offer evidence that legalized abortion has contributed significantly to recent crime reductions. Crime began to fall roughly 18 years after abortion legalization. The 5 states that allowed abortion in 1970 experienced declines earlier than the rest of the nation, which legalized in 1973 with Roe vs. Wade.

States with high abortion rates in the 1970s and 1980s experienced greater crime reductions in The 1990s. In high abortion states, only arrests of those born after abortion legalization fall relative to Low abortion states. Legalized abortion appears to account for as much as 50 percent of the recent drop in crime.

Leo Kahan, David Paton, Rob Simmons. Abortion and Crime. Voxeu.org. 10, April, 2008, Web, 22, April, 2011.

The hypothesis that the legalization of abortion contributed to a dramatic fall in crime rates in the United States, originally proposed by John Donohue and Steven Levitt in an article in 2001 and popularized by Levitt's bestselling book Freakonomics, has been the subject of close scrutiny by other academics. Until now, this scrutiny has focused on issues of measurement and statistical specification, and there have been few serious attempts to test the Donohue and Levitt (henceforward D&L) hypothesis in countries other than the United States.

In recent research, we analyze the impact of abortion on crime in England and Wales to attempt to rectify this gap in the evidence. Examining this question in the context of the UK is important for a number of reasons, in contrast to the US, in the UK, abortions are subject to mandatory reporting and, as a result, data on (legal) abortions are complete and of high quality. For the stage prior to approximately the end of the first trimester, the abortion decision and its effectuation must be left to the medical judgment of the pregnant woman's attending physician. For the stage subsequent to approximately the end of the first trimester, the State, in promoting its interest in the health of the mother, may, if it chooses, regulate the abortion procedure in ways that are reasonably related to maternal health. For the stage subsequent to viability the State, in promoting its interest in the potentiality of human life, may, if it chooses, regulate, and even proscribe, abortion except where necessary, in appropriate medical judgment, for the preservation of the life or health of the mother.

I can hardly understand the logic behind man's laws; there's always a grey area where mutilation or even murder is seen as legal according to our justice system. Unless a mother's life is in danger and a few other extreme situations such as rape or incest, abortion should be considered as a crime. To legalize murder and claim that it has a positive impact on our society is audacious and malicious.

Religious atrocity!

Female circumcision is an operation done with a community razor without Anastasia.

Young girls, some prepared, some clueless, are brought to a secluded place; where their clitoris and labia minor gets cut off. Also in most cases their vagina is sewed back up, so only a small passage is left for menstrual blood and urine.

Female circumcision is a ritual practiced by almost 40 countries around the world. It is very well known in Mali, Kenya, and 26 other countries in Africa, it is also practiced in the Middle East and Asia, it is very popular in Egypt, Oman, and Yemen. Its practitioners claim that female circumcision is a coming of age transformation from puberty to womanhood. They claim that it is religiously and culturally connected to their way of life.

Should we support religions and cultures that are degrading, demoralizing and abusive? I believe that female circumcision is genital mutilation and can be compared to rape. A minor does not have the ability to decide his or her own path of life and should not be deformed in a way that they are forever doomed by their past. Female circumcision is wrong and it should be banned worldwide.

Although it is also performed by men, genital mutilation is mostly executed by a woman on a woman, as a tradition passed along generations, from great grand- parents, to parents, to kids. This practice is dated way before the British colonial ruling in Kenya. Female circumcision is a specific type of culturally related violent abuse suffered by African women. It seems that there is a long track of violence against women in many different cultures. Sadly, they are many women defending the tradition of genital mutilation. In this article written by Joyce E. Salisbury, she explains one of the many beliefs in the origin of female circumcision: "Female circumcision was a private affair attended by the women of the family and the woman who performed the operation. In addition to ritual purity, some of the rationales for female circumcision included the reservation of chastity and the inhibition of sexual desire, but it was also thought to promote fertility and to ensure the birth of sons."

Quotation is from Greenwood Encyclopedia of Global Medieval Life and Culture by Salisbury, Joyce E.

The Holy Bible contradicts itself about the actual spiritual significance of circumcision. In Genesis 17.10 the wisdom of God says: "Every male child among you shall be circumcised. He who is eight days old shall be circumcised…the un-circumcised child shall be cut off from his people and has broken my covenant." In Cor.7.19, it states: "Circumcision is nothing and un-circumcision is nothing…" From one God to another, I wouldn't mind that extra skin right now! There is not one place in the Bible where female circumcision is mentioned at all.

In Mali, Africa, and alike many other places in the world where young girls are being circumcised, it is supposedly part of an Islamic religious culture. Many researchers have looked and no one has yet found where it is listed in the Koran as being the laws of God. They are many practices that can be referred to as cruel, such as war, slavery, oppression, prejudice, segregation, miss-education; but we can all detect the doings of man with these acts. To include God while mutilating young girls however is insanity.

There is no religious proof that circumcision in females makes them a better and faithful wife or Muslim. There are no scientific studies or research to show that these women as being more likely to produce boys. There are however many reports of pain, lack of sexual interest and feelings, and loss of soul and dignity by the women whom have undergone this ritual of female circumcision. In the book, Warrior Marks, one part of the songs they sing after the circumcision shows just how cruel this tradition is:" You thought nobody could overcome you. You said no one could stop you, but today you were held by two women. You used to make love, but that's impossible now. You used to piss well, but you will cry when you piss now. You used to walk so graciously, but now you will walk like a toad mouse." (178) Warrior Marks.

The laws to protect human rights should be applied when there is a violation of its standards. The idea of cultural rights should not include cannibalistic alike rituals such as female circumcision. This culture of female circumcision has nothing to do with God's demands, it is only a way for man to show their power, to make one subdue forcefully to their desire to control.

Throughout history women have been downgraded, mutilated or completely banish by men in their high societies. Religion has always been a tool used by powerful man to control their peers. Laws were created by kings to protect their kingdom as time went on. Cultures began to develop in churches and in discotheques at Mount Sinai and at south beach.

The pimps and the priests each have their own books and a set of rules written by God, so they say! Thy shall not have no other God but me, thy shall not steal, thy shall not sleep with thy neighbor's wife. Are these laws related to how circumcision started? Was one of these commandments written by a king whose wife slept with a servant while he was gone to war?

Circumcision is not something that is demanded by Allah and Alice Walker verifies this information in her book: “No, it’s not in the Koran, but …Africans believe it is a religious necessity, that if you are not excised you are not clean. When I told my fiancé I didn’t want to be excised, he said he would not marry a woman who is unclean and who could not be a good Muslim. Africans believe that there is no point in going to the mosque or praying if you are not excised, because you can never be a proper Muslim.” (256) Warrior Marks

There are no concrete medical or spiritual facts on any of the theories to prove that Female circumcision is helpful in any way; as a matter of fact, they are many logical reasons why this practice should be terminated. The operations are done with the same razor so if one kid has a disease all the others get it. The kids are getting impregnated at a too young age so there is a high rate of mortality. Some girls have nervous breakdown and become permanently mentally ill. Etc. One victim talks to Alice Walker in the book Warrior Marks: "Yes, my father must have known it was painful, because he knew they had to cut something off. There are young women who can't stand the pain, and he heard some of the young girls- the pain, their shouts- so he knew, but he doesn't even try to understand- he thought it was his duty and his right to do it to his daughter. My mother said a woman has to go through three ordeals in life; we must go through excision, marriage, and giving birth. Excision is a woman's destiny." (256,257)Warrior Marks by Alice Walker and Tabitha Parmar. "

Female circumcision is genital mutilation, and is insanity. It cannot be justified in any way, culturally nor spiritually. Female circumcision fits the description of the historically violent and abusive culture against women. We must put an end to female circumcision.

Indigenous Medicine!

Alternative medicine and social accommodation has long been an objective of western medicine and are largely included in our everyday lives.

There are currently a minimum of "120 drugs" that are plant based on the shelves in our pharmacies. We have "23 languages" already being taught within the social services for interpretation purposes. We have a patenting program readily available for profit so anyone with an idea can submit their discoveries for trials.

Some knowledge is still not being passed on because the indigenous people became fearful of their knowledge being stolen and patented in different names.

Though one bad apple spoils the whole bag, western medicine always had in mind to incorporate indigenous culture to make it richer for good purposes and it does. Most of our drugs are a concentrated form or a mimic of the chemicals found in plants. The licensing authorities just give them a different name while patenting. Also while under study, a drug may have a generic name, than once it is licensed it gets a different name. "Ipecac is a drug used to induce vomiting after an allergic reaction due to poisoning was made out of the substance of a plant called Cephalic ipecacuanha." Taxol is the chemical properties of a plant used to help with tumors." Many pharmaceutical companies prepare plant based drugs simply by extracting out the active chemicals from the plants. "Cynarin for example is found in artichokes and is used for liver problems and hypertension." Even when a scientist is able to make a copy a drug without using a plant, the idea still came from a plant. Well over "50% "of our known medicine came from plants.

In Africa many countries still depend on alternative medicine for most sicknesses. "Zimbabwe's government recently announced that the country had run out of the critical painkiller morphine. It was just the latest development in a debilitating health care crisis that has seen hospitals turn away patients because of drug shortages. In the absence of even a basic drug such as paracetamol, desperate patients like 44-year- old asthma sufferer Susan Pamire have turned to traditional herbs.

While traditional healers have long retained a rural client base, urban residents are now also turning to them. "Traditional herbs have become the sole alternative for me, even though I still prefer medicine from the clinic," said Pamire, who has also battled hypertension for years. Better these visits to the Inyanga [the local name for a traditional healer] than wait for tablets from the clinic, which I know are not available, or else I would die waiting, “the mother of five told IPS. Zimbabweans turn to indigenous medicine 01 March 2011 - 05:47 By SAPA, “the medical world has always been one in trying to find ways to cure diseases.”

Although researchers may have abused their power to gain money, the medical society as a whole remains a good industry. The mistakes that we've made are hopefully lessons to make us better and stronger. Cases like Lia Lee in "the spirit catches you and you fall down ", are a building block to our future and not a failure. Western medicine is an extension of indigenous medicine and it does include the medical aspects that have always existed.

If you were mine!

If you were mine, life would have been a paradise, and the sun would have shine day and night to give us warmth and light, I would not be so sad. If you were mine, time would have been fun and nice, and I would have been happy to play, the lovers rock that you like to make you feel so high.

But now my patience's almost gone, ever since the day you left me alone; you might be over it because you're strong, what about me I can't go on. Now the pain is in my bones, making me feeling a sad song. I'm like a horn which is all torn, in the back of an abandon home; singing a sad song!

If you were mine, I would not be so down and out, running around and around every town trying to find so peace of mind; my heart is crying out loud! If you were mine, I would be the good friend and companion that you've always wish to have, you would've seen when I'm fine, when I smile.

There's a black crow underneath the steps of the church!

Mom I see a shark under the bed! Pop I see a shark under the bed! A shark named Mary A shark named Mary Pearls, E,E,E,E.

When I asked the shark what him want fe eat? The shark looked at me and said, what you got fe eat? I've got beef, chicken, fish, piglets or turkey, I smiled. The shark laughed at me and said you are so funny.

A shark him na speak, not enough English, Not enough to find its way ina the shed. A shark them have teeth, but they don't have feet to walk up on to the shore and crawl under the bed.

A shark named Mary, there's a black crow underneath the steps of the church! A shark named Mary, eeee!

Well child, this girl is 6, you know they have dreams, like the broom that was talking to her from behind the door! Wisdom is in these kids, Jah knows what she means, like the wicked man stock in the cracks of the floor.

A shark under the bed have no place to hide instead must have lost its head. Telling you we must go to the mall and buy a brand new doll, today, for me to pay.

A shark named Mary! There's a black crow underneath the steps of the church.

Woman I love you

I barely knew her name, but behind her pretty eyes there was so much pain. Somebody else had broken her heart, now this girl was falling apart. Some tines it rains. Everyone is a stranger at first, but she makes me feel this loving thirst, to cool down her hurt. Be with her in good and bad. Make her smile when she's feeling sad, every day ya heard, massive have you heard?

Woman I love you, A oui I love you. Je t'aime au Cherie, I love you darling.

On the dance floor I could feel her body getting closer to me. With no amplifier, I could hear her breath talking silently, telling me, to take her home tonight, treat the girl right, dinner, candle light, love making all night.

C'est une histoire d'une fille qui revenait de paris, Oui elle etait belle et ausi loin de son pays.

I met this pretty girl by the name of Cherie, in a dance hall party near New York

City. A modern kind of girl, she was not a dibididibi; she just received a degree from a university. Ragamuffin party, this girl wants to jam with me; pushed against my body, say she wants agany. Oui this girl she's wining skill, tonight she feels love hungry, I must give her this loving feeling to fill up her every wish? What she wants is the kind to make a woman say wow. Tonight she pick it rough sweet affection tomorrow. 2 hours later near a Manhattan tower, this girl wanted I to come up, walk up, worm up under cover. Moving room in her bed room, girl a go lit a fire, I man was hot and ready to go do it in the shower. Tonight me a go right a book, me the pen she's the paper; she's the victim, me the actor, theatre fe strict lover. Give her bwa, give sister bwa trois fois, she said awawa. Make her sweat, body wet, and gymnastic girl body stretch. I man a roughneck, I go bump with her leg behind the neck. The girl stone from the bone, I must have almost broken her bottom.

Under the bridge!

Under the bridge in the mud traps, I see my friend, skinny from crack. How can I tell her, baby darling don't you do that. I've got my spliff, she's smoking crack; but she's the only friend I've got.

Under the bridge, in the homeless refuge, under the bridge, where we've got nothing to lose.

I stopped by the Camillus house, to get a meal. Then I walked up to 7th street, to pick up my weed. There she is, standing around the corner, talking to this guy in the Van, to see how much it will cost for them to get together. How can I tell her, baby darling don't you do that. I like my weed, this girl is addicted to crack; but she's the only one on sight to talk to with a light.

Forever Young!

I wish I could heal the world. I would need a certain potion, some kind of magic! What about the truth, would that be enough? Would they listen?

Sometimes it rains. They say running is too much pain. They have so little faith! They give up so easily. Are they too preoccupied with bills? Not enough time in the day? They want a magic shot or a pill! They want for someone to touch or say a magic word and cure them. They're dreaming of an afterworld, where all their sins are miraculously forgiven. It's too much work to get healthy! They're so lazy! Their standards are so low.

Imperfection is taught to be normal. Perfection is said to be unattainable because the expansion of thoughts in infinite, but if we work on something a lot and real hare, we can get close.

We pick the best out of a pack of mediocrity. Our actions are sickening, our body is filthy physically, mentally and spiritually. We hurt each other badly, than say I'm sorry. We even think war, and killing people is admissible, as long as a room of wicked congressional leaders agrees.

Now that the evil has infiltrated our homes; our kids are being brainwashed at school with bad education. We are the first to say look at these delinquent adolescents. Instead of teaching them right, we spend our taxes building prisons for them and hire more Police. Being blind ourselves, we can't see that we've led them, to this road of corruption and destruction.

We are not descendants of animals; this is the pit that our teachers dug for us. I see our world falling in a deeper hole. I see hopeless leaders encouraging this environment of madness.

Look at them after forty, completely old. Why are you following them, they're heading towards the cave. "Life is worth much more than gold". When walking or running the steps should start on the toes. Come with me! Stay forever young!

Bigger fish to fry!

I make my money on 1, 2 yo! Microphone check, for MC! In the place to be, this is New York City! You can take a bite, on my big apple! Big business! Big fried fish!

I never wait on 3. I just grab the mic and rip it, bless it, no I'll never risk it, believe it. Blink once, and I'm out gone, I'll swiftly take an inside the park run to home plate, and score easily! "By all means necessary" My mentality and philosophy, for survival, I take no prisoners. I eliminate, incinerate all not in my crew, in my view. Like in a fire I'm the extinguisher; I terminate the chain reaction on the hypocrisies that I see, every day from this society! I guess some think they have successfully suppressed all the truth; and that they can openly, teach lies and fool all the fools in this town. But here comes the block, the blockage, the brick, and the barricade, that's me stumbling down on them with a mountain of knowledge! I learned early from my Indian ancestors, way back in grammar school, I remember their anger! Now we had to live the way of the white settlers. They came from 4,000 miles and now they're making laws against other immigrants. Back then, we never had to go to college to be somebody. Instead we would live peacefully, not knowing of destruction technology! We were masters of farming, fishing and hunting! We Aztecs were doctors of every leaf, from the forest, to the ocean's reef! All of a sudden, we are seen as savages, and uncivilized. Now we are the aliens and require a passport to move around. I was born a man; I need nothing to be a man! They were English, Spanish and French speaking; screaming and celebrating this rich land, they claimed was uninhabited; firing their murderous guns at our fathers, raping our sisters and enslaving our brothers.

I never wait on 3! The past to me is history, his story! Now for me to be a useful member of this hi-tech society, I've got to wear a suit and have a degree, shave my head and praise to Jesus! Fine! I've adapted, for goodness sake! I've got to eat this garbage because you tell me to. Ok! Now enough is enough, back off alright! Don't make me start to sing "Liberte ou la mort, grenadier a l''assault"! That's the song the slaves sang, before ousting these hurtful and heartless pirates whom had invaded our land. The Nina, the Punta and the Santa Maria, we remember the names of their ships, which are when all our nightmares started. I'm trying to forgive and forget, and move on! I don't want to travel back to 1804, the year we evacuated Napoleon. So I've invested in the market. My money's getting thick, but I'm still banging in the projects. My strategy is simply fit, Go! Roll out the magic red carpet. As a ghetto superstar; my bank account is getting thicker and is the only thing that matters. My wallet is as big as Wall Street. I can fly out to my summer home to escape the winter storms. My business is flourishing so I'm on it; marketing my product, with the most celebrated athletes; making it more and more attractive to the public.

I never wait on 3! Oh, please forgive me for my arrogance; it's the nine digits on assets blinding me, not my ignorance. I purposely forget some of my values and manners, because of my interest. I'm now celebrating the west! Thug life! Hustlers! My stock is number 3 on the top ten Hip Hop R&B charts. The police are following me every day on my walks, when I ride or in my black Benz; just for driving black, I know they're keeping track, they see I'm driving a Jetta. I'm so hood, sometimes so rude! By the tilt of my baseball cap, you might be able to tell my present mood. I've got to put on these shades so I cannot see you! Haters are so jealous of me; probably want a taste of my beef stew. I know you want to ride in my brand new S.U.V. Telling your friends that you know me. If I've never drank and smoked with you! Dude, I don't know you!

I never wait on 3. Honestly, I accept the present as it is. Not understanding certain things is sometimes better for someone's well-being; especially when comprehension is impossible or useless, alike the creation of our planet. But it's easy to tell a Native apart. No one man could portray and act as if they originate from America, and were Indians and are not. So when someone talks to me about eating organically grown local food; I tell them to take the boat back home, so they could do the same. Is eating food even a subject that should even be talked about; while there is tsunamis, earthquakes, hurricanes, war, corruption, drugs, miss-education, famine, etc? Jah Rasta, lives on sugar, milk, bread, vegetables, chicken, fish and oxygen. Well, well, well! Do you know whose family stole our land, and now owns all the bad food industry? It seems to me that there is a sect who is determined to keep people's minds preoccupied with B.S, such as religious beliefs of an after world, discouraging the majority to live this life fully and happily.

I never wait on 3! If the end of the world was tomorrow, I would have no regrets. My introduction to god would be, Father, I'm a sinner, I know nothing. Please forgive me if I've done wrong! I would not have to explain he says, or she says. It would just be me with my own heart and beliefs. I accept your judgment of me God. I am prepared to love, burn in hell, or live forever in paradise. Don't bother me with nonsense; I've got a bigger fish to fry.

War!

Man you've gone far in destruction technology. Somebody mad must have shown you that way, I see! Different groups of people struggling to survive the day, Muslims in Bosnia, dem fe someplace to stay; blood in South Africa, segregation policy, some of them, dem fighting fe food, some of them are just greedy, war fe petroleum, they say fe humanity.

"You see war in the east, war in the west, war up north, war down south. It's a war, rumors of war. It's a war, a war, rumors of war."

Somebody mad wants to keep us away. Fe a Ian, a dollar, a Dutch mark; tell me why these men angry, ya seen them talking as if a few billions is not enough for the army, than they give the poor a ion, for cover up necessity.

Still, hungry bellies killing malnourish babies. Make up and mask all of them are wearing, mad these men crazy. It's unified destruction warfare in every country.

Thy shall not kill!

You shot dead a man, blood to dust for what reason! Rude broda the Don, Babylon politician; kill your brother man is not a part of this equation, who's me number one, who's the done fight fe freedom. Work! Let us try to find a new solution. In this computation, we want inclusion not subtraction. Divided men fall out but together they stand strong. Unite African man! It doesn't matter where ya from.

We shall not kill, not they shall not kill. Thy shall not steal, no; they shall not steal. You shall not commit adultery, nor have any other God than me. To satisfy their own means, man will make exceptions to what is written.

It's a shorter life around the block for man; from breathing complications. Do right, not wrong, be good, not bad; na go help the pollution, don't live in corruption, give a positive reaction. It's so hard working together. No one is doing a good job, when we are killing each other. Loving the children is the only culture which has all the rainbow colors. We can't erase the past but we can live responsibly in the present, while envisioning the future. Everyone can drift in this new vibration. Freedom is a feeling, it's a heart condition.

Can't you see that, La misma cosa que se pasa con migo, es la misma cosa que se pasa con tigo. La meme chose vous dites arrive a vous, s'est la meme chose nous disons arrive a nous. Mim bagay yo di a ki rive a you, se mim bagay la nous di ki rive a nou. The same things that are happening to you, the same things that are happening fe we too there. Unite African man; we are strong when we are one.

She's mine!

All of dem girls, they come in a full. Nice dress on, this one sure does look good, with a black silky robe, and a most beautiful red gold and green Rasta man crown; man you should have seen how she shook up a crowd of hommies with blunts, who tried to take their chance on this black queen I want.

She's mine, this girl is mine, the doggone girl is mine.

She's not just a pretty face; you could not keep up the pace of her movements. "Judge not", the way she dances is the art to bring one excitement. How she wind up her waist, who'd believe she has faith!

Rounded up in a circle, she's in shape to rock it so. All young and old follow, they know Reggae sound is a cure, so they all showed up to the rendez-vous. Freedom fighters, they're skanking. Everyone tries to duplicate, all the funky steps she takes, some do, and they do their best, than they have to take a rest. She's a butterfly girl that will not fade away. This sister and princess is the daughter of Yahweh!

Holding this mic as my hostage !

I'm taking over the stage; I grab the mic with rage. You'll be amazed, as I parade. I'm stronger than a blaze, sharper than a razor blade. I'm having a ball, I bring knowledge to all; so dock, MCs who don't seem to understand. I'm the man with the plan. I came out with a bang. Now you know just how I am living. I'm climbing up to the top of the hip hop charts. I'm taking blocks after blocks, while you're shooting your darts. I'm making money, there's no maybe or if. I'm so swift so quick. Take a sit, and take a pick on this beat, and don't say, isht, unless your style is legit. I make em move to a groove that ooze. I put a bruise on a city at a party, stating "check out my melody." I snap, as you watch me tax, I reach maximum velocity, now that's no kind of comedy. It's a tragedy for you, 1,2,3, you're out, strike out, I took out your whole damn crew. You're through, it's true, and you don't even have a clue. I stump on chump like you who try this stunt; put a bump in your head, just like you were the brand new punk. So think! Got a hint! I Ink! You just got burnt I got taller you've shrink. Now I'll turn the page to a phrase that pays.

I'm holding this mic as my hostage.

You wanna take a hit of this, but take a sit back, relax, watch me smack some whack Mc's, wanna be like me the M and M the T, the Mighty microphone technician. I destroy these boys with toys, they wanna play. I enjoy every time that I make them pay. Hear I say, get out my way, get on your knees and pray. Cuz I'll drop a couple of lyrics that can quickly make your day. Purposely, definitely make sure you see all these styles. I've got more than enough, I'm like three times rougher, I make them rush and rush, I'm about to crush. This sucker soft like fudge, tried to bug, got dogged like a frog; go and put this in your logs. No bluff, this stuff I toss made you cuff. Don't pop another puff; you'll drop just like a rock. Won't you give up, time for me to go off. I'm about to throw off a line and conclude this rhyme. I told you once already twice, keep on rolling your dice, you'll pay the price.

Ragamuffin spell!

These girls wind a hell in a ragamuffin spell, tell I man them a gone work it well. Caribbean girls them, English girls them, American girls them, African girls them.

Feel this like a hit from a black good black ganja. Jamming at a party, getting high okay I'm stone. Ya body's overcome by a gong slam from a drummer, this rhythm is addictive make them move closer to the speakers. The music put a girl in a mood of getting in the mixture. I've got the multitude of rhymes; the music has amplitude of boom. Some seeking but can't find a simple line to rock a room. Me I own storage like a cottage in the moon. Sure I own a load times a ton of different tunes.

These skilly girls controlling their hips, Twerking, winding, working on their physique. I’ve been to Carrefour, Brixton, Laval Sud but I never seen anything like that in Munich. Ragamuffin spell, is a magnet used in the Lyrics Following, well, is the important message in the music. What is justice today? Say over filled prisons, say politics! Wrong this system is wrong, Freedom is not just for the rich. Do what you want, with respect to others. Tankou ou vle, what a go on? Sa vas bien, sak pase? These English, Creole, Francais, Espanol girls, quickly smoked a spliff, in a riff, Now dem drifting, ya hear this.

Work is work!

Neglect not the present situation surrounding your life. I know it's not easy to confront the dirt around our own eyes. Every day we wake up on the wrong set of feet. We take steps that will only in the long run make us weak. We are so preoccupied with stuff; useless thoughts; things we can't prove, can't change, have no control of. Yet we fail to grant full attention to this very moment. We make big arguments out of small disagreements.

Tomorrow is not sure. Take nothing for granted. Have fun and party, love somebody. Throw away your troubles, have no sorrows. Jump into the river, splash into the sea.

The cost of living is getting higher and higher. The owners are getting richer at the expense of the workers. The private sector controls the governments. They have not changed their tactics not even by one percent. Laborers are only getting paid enough to come back to work. Every one working should earn a decent living, there's no dumb job. I see kids on the streets selling drugs and I ask and they say; work doesn't pay, and the boss treats us like dogs.

What gives you the right to take and sell everything? I was also born on this Earth. Why are you being so discriminative? Was I a step child at birth? Why are you so scared of me? I know your history. You've been doing wrong for so long. Are you worried about retaliation?

Father we work!

Father we work but we na get no pay. Jah Jah we work but we na get no pay.

I'm talking to this thug, he says he just ran out of buds. I needed to make a trade; I got to the pawn shop too late. It's been over ten years, since I've last used this Karaoke; my hommie says he ain't got no deals, the tape recorder ain't green. So I proceeded to the next corner, hustlers slinging for dollars, I'm hungry but my hunger hurts far less than my soul. At least if I could smoke a spliff, I may fall asleep. I would pray that tomorrow, I'll get back on my feet. Can't let go of my dreams, I don't wanna grow up. I'm always gonna be a kid deep inside my heart. I've been working so hard, still, I still can't get far. I'm trying as hard as I can, something must be holding me back. I thought as long as I worked, I would not have to eat dirt.

I'm condemned to be poor; I just cannot get a break. I should have stayed in school, instead of chasing these skirts. My mom thinks I'm a fool, well, did she lose her faith? You need a working plan man, so the bills can get paid. I'm learning to be a man mom, she said the rent just got raised. I did everything I could to give you intelligence, boy. You chose to clean the earth, well is it that important? You could've been a doctor, like your sister Chantee, or even a buffalo soldier, like your brother Dj.

Father we work but we na get no pay. Jah Jah we work but we na get no pay.

In the Ghetto!

I saw them as they stepped out of the labor pool van, sweaty and dirty as they walked their way into the inside corner of the convenient store to cash in, the worth of one day of labor. Forty eight dollars for eight hours of hard work, before taxes; I heard one of them say, madam! Would you please give us, three orders of that jerk chicken and rice; and please put a lot of gravy and spice? Yes sir, she replied! On the far side isle, that's where you'll find that bottle of Sysco, and the six pack of Coors. Yeah man! Right around the corner, that's where the brothers got the bigger sacs of Indo, just to let you know. They sat down across the street, under a tree, peacefully, to eat a warm meal, smoke a spliff, and drink some beers. They were giggling and laughing, you know!

But in the Ghetto, the people, they get brutalized. In the Ghetto, you see police patrolling all the time.

Out of nowhere! The beast came bomb rushing, handcuffing, and mishandling these poor innocent men. In a few minutes, they were gone, taken to prison; to be encaged behind bars like animals.

They are some acts committed, that a man deserves to lose his freedom, and or be put on retention. On the other hand, they are laws that are only enforced on minorities. They are a lot of petty acts that this system is calling crime, that are not truly so; but through corrupted governments we are living hell with the present laws.

It is naive to ask the devil to be righteous! We need to be humane and fair to each other. Like crabs in a bag, most of our downfalls are black against black crimes. We must have equal rights and justice. It's a struggle because Po-po is malicious.

Dance!

I am not like that child, who cheats and lies, I don't want to make you cry! Now we don't see rewards, now thing are hard, I only want to see you smile.

We can make love all night, we can dim down the lights, and dance! Sex might flourish with a life, it’s got to be just right, and we cannot take a chance.

We were only supposed to dance. Use a jimmy boy, before you get the joy. We can't romance without safety. I would love to have a baby, but I don’t have child support money when things go south and we file for divorce. Girl let's wait till we're more ready.

The money was in the bank, uncle Joe got a habit; now there ain't a brown cent. How did Uncle Joseph get the code to the credit card? Silence in the small tent, they said that grandmamma feinted, the landlord said he wants eviction or rent!

You look good baby doll! Looks don't impress me at all. Do you work at the mall? Are you a nurse who's on call? I like the sex but even more, I need a friend who's down by law. I've been in lust many times before, now It's your love I'm asking for

Melanie!

Thirteen trips, 13 buckets of water, to and from the river. Breakfast and lunch and dinner, she ironed all clothes before supper.

Even though Polo woke up this morning, with a fever; the schedule goes on!

They called her a maid, but she was a slave. Mom! I'm not a slave. They called her a maid, Oye, she was a slave. Mom! I'm not a slave.

For her to stay in that home, for food and shelter, school must be never. Way too much work around, work to be done, she's got no time for pleasure. The family will have company later, so this house must look much cleaner. Even though my brother Polo woke up this morning with a fever; the schedule goes on.

They love to abuse. When you try to refuse, they'll kick you; they’ll push you, and leave you with the bruises. When you're a retired slave, they see you as a threat, they're afraid you will teach freedom to the rest of the slaves.

Fancy Dribbling!

I see them passing by, trying not to be late for the work out. I see them rushing through, trying their hardest to get down to the park. Is it faith to say, last Sunday night, live on channel 7, I was banging your man.

This homeboy looks me in my eyes, wondering what am I gonna do next! I'm gonna take one step, bounce this ball, and dunk it in your face man! What! I'm up 2 man. That was you reacting, too late as I shoot man. I took them, two main, so called best defenders in the highest league man. You wear fatigues man? I should man. I'm like a sniper, itchy fingers on the trig man. You left me free behind the three, it's like a sure thing. Like a camera with a zoom man, I'm like boom man. Done with, Down nets, and the Knicks man, no Celtics on my truce man, no heat for my juice man, I grab a hornet and turn it into a Bobcat, I make a wizard out of a buck. I take no bull suns. I travel at a supersonic speed man. You would think I'm thunder. Game over, move over, spur me from the clippers, I blaze rockets, too fast for you pacer. Yes, like magic, I just took your nuggets.

Do you know Nicholson? Have you seen Don Pereon? You're a Laker! Ah! Now I understand why you're so bad, it's all in the bag. I'm threatening, shuffling, off balance, you are, stumbling. Now I'm muscling, spring-idling, Rim-ironing. Call me cook, you just got shocked. You ankle is on the recipe for my basketball soup. Poof! Another one spooked by the fancy dribbling.

Truly! Y , y ,y, y, reggae music a de Don!

You're a musician? Part time man. That's why you heard the dribble sounded like a drum set. I'm a prophet, you're the puppet, when I bounce next, Simon says you dance left, now right! I didn't say Simon says, the ball was already passed before your last breath! MRI test! Fractured tibia, broken ulna! He tried to guard me solo. I'm like oh! No. Disrespect, you'll regret it. I'm ecstatic; you've made a curse wish. You got me all upset, now did I not tell you so, I can't be dealt with? You're a non-believer. Impostor you must be served with the twist now! You're kind of tall, let's play slip and fall, here's the ball. Now you see it, now you don't. G-alert! G-alert! This is an emergency; call time out, change strategies. Poof! Spooked, you just got took. Your dignity is on the picture for my newest web site post Cooked by the fancy dribbling.

Alcohol is a poison!

Alcohol depletes the oxygen supply to the brain; that's why you feel dizzy and lose instant reflex capabilities. Alcohol is the underlying cause of many chronic diseases. The propaganda that one drink or two is good for you is misleading.

Since it is legal to drink and there is so much profit; the big heads get together to continue their lies and involvement in insanity. I care not what the research says. I've made my own research and studies of alcohol. My body mind and soul feel better without. My lungs and my liver are working so much better without alcohol. I run faster, longer, without getting tired. The source that made the studies on alcohol, and said it was okay to drink was biased.

How can a sick person determine when someone is well? How could there be any objection to the top choice of legal drug to the elite class.

Also the words used to promote red wine are so carefully chosen. "In moderate quantity" "one or two glass a day". Just like "one aspirin a day". Anything that you do on a daily basis becomes habitual. I smoke weed, so I say, one joint a day, to keep the devil away. I've been too high and low places; when it's your drug of choice, you'll say anything to defend it.

Fair Treatment!

Will there ever be such morality in America? Fair Treatment; where all man is treated equally. Are we blindfolded, can't you see, we are still dealing with the old Roman laws. We will always be seen by him as a less capable human being, and as a second class citizen.

Inside America, the colonial rules and regulations still apply: "The slave has no right to retaliate, he has no right to refuse, his property can be taken, his wife and his kid, and nothing is to be done to the assailants."

My family is from New York, Boston, home of the 54th, 9th, 10th and 369th Regiments. We gave our lives freely, maybe stupidly for the freedom of white America. Never once in our existence, were we given our fair share of respect and ransom.

Fair treatment! I want my 40 acres that my ancestors were promised, now. Justice and Freedom for all! Are we dreaming? As I was playing homeless, I have trod through the many cities in the United States. I intentionally remained righteous to see if it meant anything. America's treatment of me shows that slavery is simply more technological. Blacks are targeted so most of our youth cannot reach certain levels in society.

Just like we were only called upon when the going got rough during all the past wars. When will we open our eyes to see, that we are being used, that we are still a commodity They see most of us as a labor force, good only for their domestic needs.

Our strong muscles have built the Great America! Why can't we find our home? Where are our moms? Why can't we build our own nation? Why can't we take care of our own?

Abraham Lincoln was murdered for daring to stand for humanity, so has Dr. King, and Malcolm, and Mr. Marley, and Peter tosh, and Ti Manno; and so has anyone who dared to stand up for black liberty. Haitians, Jamaicans, we don't like slave masters, Jah know.

I have in me the blood of Haitian Grenadiers and Jamaican Maroons, trodding through Babylon as a buffalo soldier. I am not afraid; I will not accept the continuing enslavement and the unjust treatment of my people.

The Klu Klux Klan has long infiltrated in the Police and the American government and they hate our black skin. They have liquor stores in every corner in our neighborhood. They facilitate the drug and gun trade to reach our youth, than the same ones snitch out to the Police to come get us.

The athletes and entertainers are the only ones partially accepted in America. Most of them with millions however, invest in the same system that is oppressing their own kind; Or else they get set up by a white girl and their money gets taken away.

I have voluntarily, blindly, stupidly served this country; I thought it was my duty to the place where I was born. I am slowly beginning to regret the sweat I have shed for this land. No matter how far we have gotten with this fake democracy. We will never be considered American.

Remember always that you are an African-American; and there will never be fair treatment here for you. Justice, freedom and liberty is a human right. "L'union fait la force, United we're strong." I care not for this slow progress. "Black progress” I want it now. We can build our own leagues. Stand up for fair treatment, equal rights and justice.

Black VS Black!

On and on and on to the ding ding dong; black division this is the mighty microphone technician on a mission. This selection is about freedom. We’re searching for peace, or some kind of liberation. At this rate of hate, this race needs to consolidate; No need for debate, wait, I’ll elaborate. Black against black is weak, weak whack. These words that I’m speaking are not simply a rap. Don’t turn your back; I’ve got the right to state that fact, America’s for whites, but black against black is the knife in the rate of our mortality. You claim you’re strong, maybe stone, should be thrown, in the dumpster, find your partner; yeah you're a full time sucker. It's in my thoughts, but you would not understand or comprehend; why we are not friends, because you're so damn insane. It is simple and plain our brain doesn't work on cocaine. But you've got to do, what you've got to do. You don't like what I'm saying than check this. It's nothing new from me to your stupid crew. You ain't S.H.I.T, in my books.

And I hate it I admit, how can I explain, It is such a shame; you're the one to blame for. Bullet holes on a brother's soul, he was blown, He felt so damn numb. Bullet holes on a brother's soul who was blown. It's not the bullet or the gun; it was the man who pulled the trigger who was so damn dumb. Black against black is weak weak whack. Black against black is weak weak whack.

I express myself, something good for your health, in just one breath; I was this close to death. I live four inches from hell, a few seconds to these gun shots. I was born with a spell, growing up around my block. I'm always on the edge, like I'm stepping on a thin line. I knew a guy named Feze; I remember this with clear mind. It was not Halloween night; he didn't even have a mask on, he looked like the devil's son, He would love to make me numb, for my money or for fun. He said hold up, it's a stick up, give it up; before I bust your book learning cells out. I wasn't scared because I'm good at karate; He was fat as a pig so I said come and get it. I hit him with a fist, out came four of his teeth, I followed with an elbow he coughed O hell no; he pulled out his nine and said, "Meet my little friend." I don't know Shao Lin God damn it, ain't got no time to play kung Fu my man. Bang blagada, bang, bang, I was blown, I felt so damn numb.

Don't call me your bro, because I go with the flow; Dropping mystic lyrics on dope tempos. You're not a bro, you're a foe, so let go, of that green black and red, you might as well be dead; because just for some blow, you committed a crime. You had no flow, and you needed a dime. You've lost your mind, when you triggered your nine, another victim was blown for a couple of pounds; how does it sounds, you've just emptied your rounds, on an old man a black man, a good man with nothing but giggling change for his children. You popped him once, twice, that wasn't nice; but you're so, so blind, you can't see with your eyes, for the simplest prize, you'll sick a man till he dies. You're not wise, you don't realize. You've got to have it, I don't buy it, and you've just got a habit for that crack hit. You needed a fix dose so you could keep cool; killing for material things you're only a fool. Our people won't find freedom until you follow these rules. You've got to stop, destroying your own. Were baptized in blood? You're the son of a gun. Do you call that fun? Watching another life blown, feeling numb!

Avez Maria!

Je vois tous ces malins, hypnotizes par leurs vins. Cette vie sans conscience, qui ne donne point la main. Au petit geant et a la petite princesse. Qui n'ont pas de maison, il n'ont pas d'education, Ils n'ont memes pas du pain. Mais comment allez.

Alleluia, avez, Maria, dormez- vous? Reveillez-vous! Allez.

Tout autour des grandes villes, l'on ne sais plus, qui est fils ou filles. Ils sont tous perdu, l'argent est la malice qui les a vaincu. Ils ne raisonnent plus. Mais non ici, ils n'ont pas le bon Coeur, qui donne a la terre, Le meilleur de soi meme. Comment Eve, n'ai je pas payer pour cette affaire, sur la croix, a Jerusalem.

Mais Gate!

Mais gate,se pa tout mange, ki se repa, ke diab la ka manje roye. Mais gate, Yo di pitimi pa kon gate, min gin treze repa, se manje rangj yo ye roye. Mais gate.

Mrin prale nan kafou la croi, devan baron samedi soi, Mrin pral illiminin baleine oye. 6 baleine noi, mrin semente 7 foi, mrin pral intepele, tout 101 loi yo.

Mais gate. Mrin pral trace, shema, nan kafou 4 point, moun ki pas rimin se pou yo pedi voi yo. Mais gate. Tet kabrit fin coupe, sang mete nan cui, mrin pral sevi temoin, mete offrande nan coin. Mrin di papa Ogou,se pitit Ezili Freda. Moun ki pa met main nan main, jete yo bay damballa.roye.

Ti gasson ap joue mab, toute ti fam pou yo joue cay, gran moun ap boue clerin, loi pale lang nan nin. Moun ki pa vle rimin. Pran maladi serin. Se pou ke yo sispane bat la roye.

I'm a nigger

She likes it when I act like a fool, but her daddy thinks showing off my back crack ain't cool. I'm a rude boy with friends and money for bail, jealous f,,..kers spent the whole year trying to send me to hell. O, you think that I'm bad, I thought you liked me because I could ball, I tried get big to please you more than any other guy. O, no, you think that I'm odd; I thought you would love me, if I was hardcore, so I tried to get up on my hustle as an answer in reply.

I know, she loves me, cuz I'm a nigger, I'm a nigger. Good god, I know that he hates me, cause I'm a nigger, I'm a nigger. I don't drink, but I'll buy her a 40oz, cuz I'm a nigger, I'm a nigger. Oakland's got the Dubs, I know cause I'm a nigger, I'm a nigger. I ain't mad at you cuz, I'm a nigger, I'm a nigger. Don't be so mad at me, cause I'm a nigger, I'm a nigger. I ain't scared of you dogs, cuz I'm a nigger, I'm a nigger. Don't be so scared of me, cause I'm a nigger, I'm a nigger.

Although some other guys thought she was poison, O, I had 3,6,9 good reasons to keep her tight on one limb. In spite of the fact that she knew I was trouble, ish just seem to follow me everywhere I go. But now she's getting blasted, her mind is twisted.

Typical California girl, she likes to ride in my Mack truck, she likes the big rocks. Powder up her nose as if she was eating donuts, got every other man she knew bankrupt. In the elevator, she edges on dangerous behaviors. She enjoys the thrill of being watched by other cats and dogs; when the door opened up, she was still making out with the local drug dealer.

She can act like a sweet flower and then turn the hot water off to give you a cold shower. Be very, very careful her thongs, she can be so candylicious, but her habits are serpentine with a high percentage that is all so very venomous.

She says I don't care what you think; I'm gonna be me regardless. No matter what I do, right or wrong, you would still complain and find something to cause me stress and malaise. Anyway, go ahead and keep on xxxxxxx with me each and every day, with a brand new different law you've just passed. One of these nights, I'm gonna lower my standards and change my religion a bit, hit the Grey Goose to help me get loose, and xxxx both of you in the xxx; and it's all legal, for sure!

The rainbow and the moon!

What in the world would make you think that you are better than me; I don't know why you say that you are better than me! Is it because your skin is pale, and you got keys to the jail cell? Is it because you have money and weapons, and connections to bend the law? Is it because you're a murderer, and you are patrolling, hidden behind the badge, looking for reasons to take me to prison?

I see you wearing your shades of war, driving in your mad a gas car. You'd like to think you're a star, but I know who you are. You ain't better than me. You're no better than. You are not better than me, oh no, not at all.

You tried to camouflage the fact that you don't like me at all, and you've succeeded for so long. I'm just here doing my thing, but you always claim that I'm thugging. Maybe you know the situation you've put me in, you're surprised. You hope that I fall in your traps.

I'm a man of great patience, I think twice before I act. "You won't miss your water, until your well runs dry." (Marley) I'm a rainbow too you know. I don't think you're better than me. You are not better than me, not at all.

In love with you!

I'm in love with a world, so young, so dumb and so ungrateful. Yes, I'm in love with you, so blind, so unkind. You're always on time. You're so up to date, so in style, so realistic.

I see so many sick from lack of education. But instead of prevention for a sustainable solution; we chose to build more prisons and create more medication.

Is it good parenting; when you don't have money for gas you should borrow? Is that a realistic mental state, to teach the parents of tomorrow? Was it not you yesterday, the minister of education? Is this your solution; those who don't agree with your insane mentality, to put them all in detention? Isn't this your man made war and paradise? Isn't this your corruption?

You're looking pretty in your suits and ties? Is this what you call civilized; a society only to satisfy your own mind? You are not related to an animal; why are you acting like a cannibal? How can you take pleasure in establishing sorrow; you can never destroy the hope for tomorrow!

I'm in love with you. Yes my heart beat in pain, my head feels like in a blaze, my pen shouts the hails, and I can't find the rails. I'm in love you with you, ooh, oh you all!

And my heart beats the pain, my head kicks the aches, my ink writes the tales, my feelings are in a craving, and I can't find smooth sailings. I'm in love with you, ooh, oh you in the mirror!

I'm in love with you. Ooh, ooh, you too ooh, oh you all. I'm in love with you.

.

Glory!

Glory to Jah! I give Jah, all the glory. Glory to jah! Give Jah glory.

The life I live is alike the one of the offspring of Zion. The love I need is from a friendly companion. The joy I seek is that smile on their faces. The wealth I need is a peaceful happy place.

It touched me inside when you've told me you love me. It broke my heart when I realize that you don't really care. It's half the job that you recite a few prayers. It doesn't mean much that you're attending a church.

So much has been said, but a little bit done. They're still destroying jah children by the million. Yet until the philosophy, of his Imperial majesty, king highly Si-La-Si, is accomplished, Earth will not know peace.

I see through you!

The alliance is married to wrong. It is still the same sharks today, who were at the helm of the old Roman Empire! With a well-organized human farm; a number of selectees, desperate and hungry, have to work through the doors of immigration! Most immigrants are good, law abiding, hardworking citizens, and seeking opportunities in faraway lands. They find themselves trapped in the concrete jungle, being classified as burden, boat people or even criminals!

I see through you! You hate to see me make it everywhere I go. After all the wrong you've done to me. I still came through! I see through you! I'm gonna take care of my people; I want my own key combination to the cargo. I see through you! You know I'm laughing at you! Although you thought I would be mad at you.

When I see the brutal tactics being utilized today by governments, the international laws might as well not exist if they were meant to advise Santo Domingo.

No denying this is the continuing land of hypocrisy. There is no diplomacy; therefore there isn't any democracy without money and weapons. Inside the market place, racism and favoritism make women have to sell their body and their soul to advance.

The situation is no different in America, colored people are being oppressed and placed in second class neighborhoods; as we are patrolling the world claiming to be fighting for democracy!

I must be dreaming, I thought we were free. Free at last! Now I see, it was just a dream. As I trod through the streets of Babylon analyzing how the system keeps us down.

Il est trop tard!

Il est trop tard pour s'inquiter, dans le passe il n'y a que des heroes. La vie a ces bons et mauvais temps, comme si c'etait un rollercoaster qui nous emmenait tous zero a zero.

Je veux t'aimer, il est trop tard pour que se soir, que tu dois t'en aller. Il est trop tard, je ne veut plus de memoire de ce qui s'etait passé hier, pretes moi tes charmes, aide moi donc a tout oublie.

Je veux t'embrasser pour renouvler notre recontre. Restons amis, avec interests, on est trop grand pour re-arrange nos mauvaises manieres et nos vieux sentiments. J'espere bien que tu m'entends, il est trop tard pour perdre la patience. Laisse moi te faire chante comme une Pipirit. Je voudrais tant etre jelee, et toi biscuits.

Super Modelle!

Je ne connais meme pas assez de mots dans mon vocabulaire en Francais, pour te dire Mamamia, combien je t'aime. Non, je n'ai pas etudie dans les grandes universites; je n'ai aucun degree en psychologie pour exprimer l'effet de te voir sourire pret de moi dans cette heure. Tout ce que je sais! Resens tu la chaleur? C'est bon, tu ressembles etre contente et mouiller dans la sueur. Le touché s'electrifie sur nos coeurs!

Elle est une super modelle. Elle a un talent d'apporter la joie pour un moment et instantanement vous faire vivre le Bonheur d'un reve dans une magazine. Elle est une super modelle.

L'as tu vue hier. Descendant du Limo; le chauffeur auvre la porte. Tous les cameras flash, et tous les journalist la raporte. Vous ne saurez jamais qu'elle est timide, quand elle me parle après minuit. Se ne sont pas simplement ses souliers, ses accessories ou ses vetements qui lui font belle. J'aime son coeur vivid, et sa facon de faire plaisir.

Quand la pluie tombe!

Quand la pluie tombe, elle ne comblera pas seulement un hombre. Quand la pluie gronde, elle eclaircira tout le monde." When the rain falls, it won't fall on just one man's house."

Le cinema m'a fait connu, plutot comme un servant sans valeur. La facon du maître d'esclave m'a battu, pour jouir de ma sueur et rire de ma douleur. D'ou viens cet gars avec son menteau tout vers, s'est il perdu, pensant que la mort me fera peur. Ce livre doit etre vecu; je ne suis qu'un pond du lion qui est le roi et l'auteur.

Je crois en Dieu, mais je ne suis pas un home d'eglise. Je n'adore pas le feu, mais j'utilize les scriptures. Attends mon vieux, ne cours pas si vite contre le mur. Il n'a uncune sensation. Cette bariere n'a pas d'oreille; son cerveau est dans ces pieds, pour le briser, il faut percer sa foundation. La raison n'est point le but d'un home ignorant.

I'm gonna love you!

I've got to get rid of this nightmare, when I saw you standing way over there sad, and I couldn't hold you in my arms to keep you warm. I'll try to hide it, but I have fear, if I push too hard when I lay it down, I'll make a big mistake and lead you on. The truth is, damn girl, damn it you turn me on.

I'm gonna love you, I'm gonna love you, I'm gonna love you.

I want to have you on the phone, saying you miss me so bad. I would speed through rush hour from hustling to come rub your back. You've been working so hard to show love to this Earth. It's funny how wicked man can make you run out of breath, and bring you down to get you to swallow your words.

In the crib!

I still believe in Santa Claus, and Rudolph, the red nose rain deer! If I am dreaming, please don't wake me up, cause I do, I want to be lost! We were celebrating, screaming and singing Christmas carols; gifts bought and borrowed.

Spark up the ease, open the ish, and turn the volume up, in the crib. I could hear them singing, the jingle bells ringing, what a special feeling, in the crib! They were celebrating, at the top of their tongues screaming, this baby is the king, in the crib!

Young and older than ten; they were playing pretend the holy baby had re-appeared! Ready or not, twenty go! Here I come! My heart is the sword of love! My feet are the stamp of truth! One of me versus a world flooded with corruption; still no contest for a fighter from the envoy of Zion! My faith is Iron! I am a lion!

Leve!

Mande map mande sa kap fet la, nattydread, Rasta,dreadlock.

Leve, kampe, mache, pale. paye Baron Sam dil map pase la. Leve, tout moun se terre tounin nan terre. Sa-ou pa konin, pi gran pase-ou. Leve.

Dlo rivie tojou sot nan sous. Tout moun ap presse tankou yo te nan kous. Gade sou tet etage-a wa we un gros bous, tanpri, ale achte deux grin citron pou tousse.

Mete chemise blanc pounal mache nan parade, Carotuou boule devant tout embasad. Rocket ap tire tankou se guerre nan Bagdad, mon cher gade ou pa we se ou paket moun malad.

Colombus get ta mere,Kaka zoreil gyn gou amer. E si ke ou paka we claire, Buddah pa kon mete lunettes de vue mon frere.

Monche ro pa kimbem nan fouk, fe ou ti lachem poum ka pran souf. Mim si ou te tande loi te kon mache sou clou. Sa pa vle dil ka pran kle kou.

Gade kijan yo tue ti Martin, ou mange chaud yo bal nan main, sa se mechanste. Yape tue jeneusse nou kou chien. Gele yo blie ke nou se moun Benin. Tale na lumin baleine noi nan bouda yo, mim sin pa gyn balles na lage zange loi baleine fe regle ave yo.

Yo no soy Capitalist!

No es realistico, que una persona tiene todos, y un otra nada y mas! Por treinte anos elle se va a trabajar. Por una semana se sentir enferma, y perdida toda que tal! La policia muerta su esposo, porque ello estaba un negro que vivir a Dominicana! Ella tiene tres chicanos que necessitan comida; para buscar su apartemente, ella se vas a la calle en la nocho para prostitutionar.

Como se dice que es libre, es siempre porque tiene dinero y un checke. Adonde vivir en el ghetto es un guerilla normnal cuanto viene la noche. Ella esta a su casa cansado, porque ayer un vagabond se fue con su pulsa. No tiene dinero para partir, no esta fuerte para courir, Tiana se resignado despues mourir.

Los corporations destructaran la tierra, se vayan como un pierra, como no hace un corazon o cabessa. Dentro la malediction, el hombre se vas con un semi-automatic, como un inundation del malo vivo en su cuerpo. Dice que es un republic democratic, pero no visto el amor o la sympathia para todo los pueblos. Los pobres estan en el mismo prison, con los que se dicen criminales.

Yo no soy un hombre malo, yo no soy contentado con la situacion de nosotros probrecimos. Soy un player mad problematic, cuanto entrar en el politic, pero yo no soy un fantasist, yo no soy capitalist.

Tears!

Tears, tears, falling all over my face. Tears, tears, now my mouth knows the taste. Tears, tears, falling all over my face. Tears, tears, now my heart knows the taste.

Tear drops, falling all over my face; I remember this used to be the place, where we used to share, so much love. Now love is gone, tears is the theme to our song, pain has entered our home, tell me, where is happiness?

Tear drops, falling all over my face, memories of our own little place, where we used to share so much love. Now everything is wrong, tears is the chorus to our song, anger is the theme in our songs, tell me, where can I find happiness?

The question mark!

What is our limit? What is infinity? What is eternal life? Can our bodies live forever? Is death the beginning of an end? Is life partial? How long has good and evil coexist? Is it logical to try and separate right and wrong? Does everyone see good and bad differently? Did Jesus conquer death? Why do I see him on a cross? What is the Catholic Church trying to teach us? Does a person only see God and heaven when they are dead? Is it because we have no proof of life after death? Does every man have a heart? Do men only think with their mind? Do they only see with their eyes? Is it the job of evil to misdirect us? What is love? Is love a composition of hope and fear? Can it be unconditional? Does it always have some kind of attachment? Is it petty to celebrate grits for dinner? Is it vanity to only want fish? Are we preoccupied with too many demands? Why are they any children hungry? Am I asking too many questions? Who knows all the answers? Who is to blame? Who can we trust? Where are he and she? Is he you and me? God, would you please send me an answer?

Acupressure is the theory which helps to mold our body, mind and soul by using the hands as a surgical tool to focus on our body. Working through painful situation has its gain; if the negative energy can be harvested to enrich our knowledge. This is only a road for the strong and the brave. This is a book for seekers of the unknown.

It is easy to unite in war and destroy in anger. But to fix the problem, which is to correct the flaws in ourselves; it takes strength and tolerance, courage and perseverance. So we prefer to serve bug wine and annoyingly cheese others, than to work inside our own home, family and shelter.

Thank you! To all souls whom have helped me grow. I was told that wisdom was more conductive than silver and gold; so share with me this pot of info. When walking or running, the steps start with the toes, use both sides equally.

You have read the thesis. Proof read under microscope and endorses it. Try it and analyze it. Don't stay too long on the superficial, grammatical and vocabulary errors. Don't be so vain. Walk with me side by side. I need not any followers. No one can feel your pain, no one can walk or breathe for you, no one can save you but yourself. We can work together.

I love Earth, I love you all. I love to ball; and make boutique calls. No one is coming to the all-night party; unless we unite for the better, we all will fall deeper into this age of war.

I think I own the world; I bit the apple, the poison is in my blood, I feel as if it's my duty to fix it. I am also responsible for its state.

By consuming parts of my knowledge in rehabilitating the human body; you would have acquired the wisdom of old. Practical sports medicine is my experience with Dexter Scoliosis, along with the sweat of my thoughts which have turned into honey and sweet love of health. Acupressure is the answer to physical health; which will in turn enhance our mental and spiritual understanding of the human. Learn how to walk, like in the years before a child can clearly speak. Ink is sometimes more powerful than fire coming out of a dragon's teeth.

Alain Rousseau/researcher

beanjah@gmail.com, facebook.com, twiter.com, google.com

References

1. Depression. (2012). In Encyclopedia Britannica. Retrieved from http://www.britannica.com/EBchecked/topic/158349/depression

2. King, Laura, A.Ph.D, The science of psychology: an appreciative view, 1st Ed, p539.

3. The Utilization of Antidepressants and Benzodiazepines among People with Major Depression in Canada. Chiranjeev Sanyal, BPharm, MSc1; Mark Asbridge, PhD2; Steve Kisely, MD, PhD3;

Ingrid Sketris, PharmD, MPA (HSA)4; Pantelis Andreou, PhD5.The Canadian Journal of Psychiatry, Vol 56, No 11, November 2011,p667.

4.Clemmitt,M.(2009,June 26). Treating depression: Is effective treatment available. Vol 19,Issue 24, Retrieved from http://library.cqpress.com/cqresearcher/

5.Worsnop, R. L. (1992, October 9). Depression. CQ Researcher, 2, 857-880. Retrieved from http://library.cqpress.com/cqresearcher/

1. Warrior Marks by Alice Walker.

1. World Health Organization

www.ingramcontent.com/pod-product-compliance
Lightning Source LLC
Chambersburg PA
CBHW051909170526
45168CB00001B/305
* 9 7 8 1 5 1 5 3 0 3 9 8 5 *